THE COMPLETE
PLANT-BASED COOKBOOK
FOR BEGINNERS

250+ QUICK, DELICIOUS AND WHOLESOME RECIPES

WITH 21-DAY MEAL PLAN FOR PLANT-BASED DIET

RICHA D'CRUZ

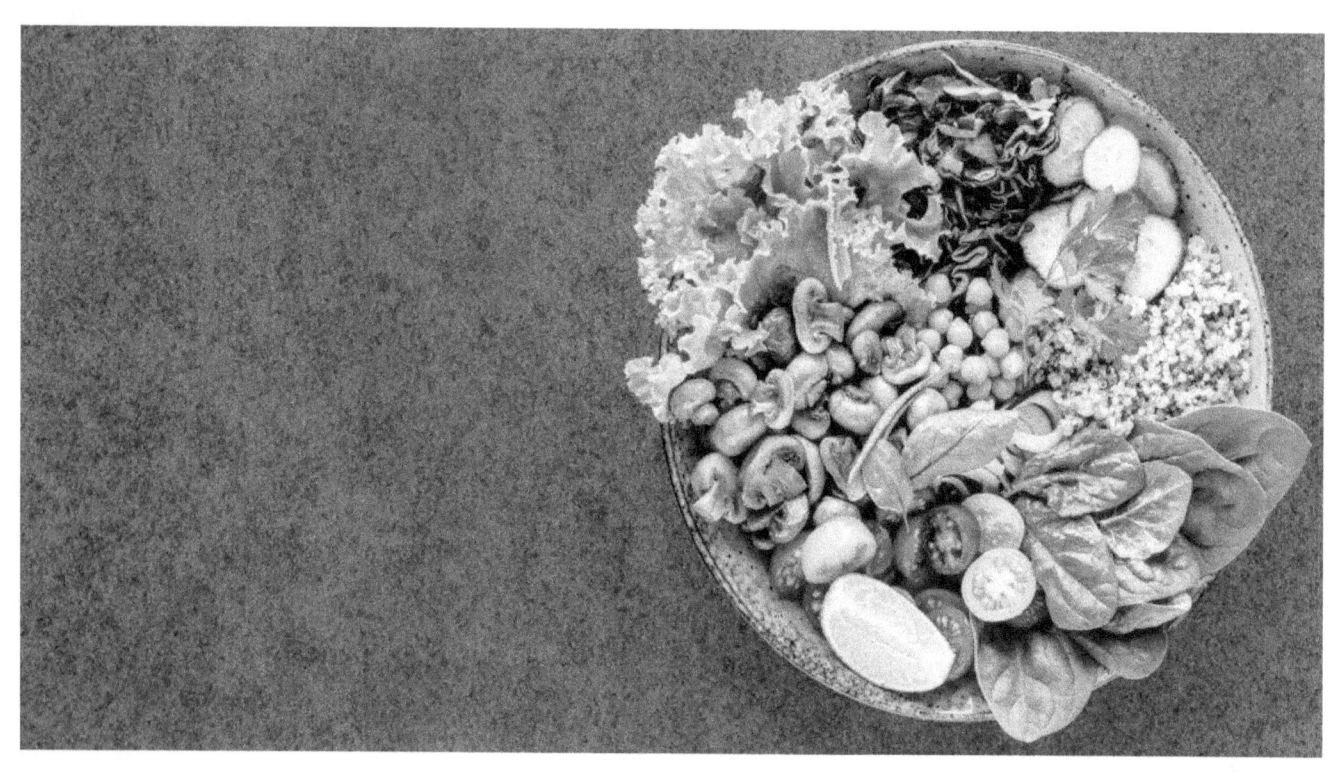

Copyright © 2020 by Richa D'cruz

All rights reserved.

No part of this publication may be reproduced, distributed, or transmitted in any form or by any means, including photocopying, recording, or other electronic or mechanical methods, without the prior written permission of the publisher, except in the case of brief quotations embodied in critical reviews and certain other noncommercial uses permitted by copyright law.

For permission requests, write to the publisher, addressed "Attention: Permissions Coordinator," at the address below.

Printed in the United States of America

1. The main category of the book — Vegan Cooking (Books)

2. Another subject category — Vegetable Cooking

3. More categories — Weight Loss Recipes

First Edition- December, 2020

Contents

Introduction 12
    Allowed food on a plant-based diet? 12

Basic Ingredients and Shopping List 13
    The 5 Basic Pillars of the Plant-Based Shopping List 13

Chapter 1 16

Breakfast 16
    Avocado Toast 16
    Vegan Pancakes 17
    Chocolate Oatmeal 18
    Vegetarian Tacos 19
    Instant Oats 20
    Vegan Bread 21
    Sweet Potatoes Toast And Blueberries 22
    Pasta With Lemon, Asparagus And Cauliflower 23
    Zucchini Rolls Stuffed With Dried Tomato Paté 24
    Vegetable Seasoned Oats 25
    Vegan Pea Burger 26
    Vegan Tart 27
    Oatmeal With Chia Seeds 28
    Peanut Butter Pancakes 29
    Vegetable Quiche 30
    Black Bean Flutes 31
    Soy Milk And Oatmeal Smoothie 32
    Vegan Omelette 33
    Pecan Butter 34
    Rice Cakes 35
    Oatmeal Pancakes 36

Chia Vegan Pancakes 37
Oatmeal Porridge 38
Chia Banana Porridge 39
Blueberry Buckwheat Pancakes 40
Oatmeal Soaks With Goji Berries 41
Liquid Nutrition Smoothie 42
Oatmeal Pancakes With Honey and Strawberries 43
Protein Smoothie of Pear, Apple And Banana 44
Smoothie of Pear And Banana 45
Pineapple Kefir Smoothie 46
Green Smoothie With Fruits and Vitamins 47
Granola, Greek Yogurt And Red Berries 48
Waffles With Peanut Butter 49
Chia And Mango Pudding 50
Papaya Juice, Grapefruit And Nopal 51
Avocado Sandwich And Spinach 52
Hummus And Avocado Cream 53
Portobello Tortilla 54

Chapter 2 55

Soups & Stews 55

Cabbage Soup 55
Sprouted Lentil And Brown Rice Stew 56
Corn And Jalapeno Soup 57
Red Pepper Cream Soup 58
Pumpkin Soup 59
Corn Chowder 60
Nopales Soup 61
Vegetables Broth 62
Green Soup 63
Simple Vegan Miso Soup 64
Zucchini Cream With Tofu 65
Carrot Cream With Ginger 66
Red Lentil Hummus Cream 67

Homemade Vegan Mayonnaise 68

Cauliflower Cream And Coconut Milk 69

Split Pea Soup Recipe 70

Noodle soup with broccoli and ginger 71

White Garlic Soup 73

Butternut Squash And Black Bean Chili 74

Sweet Potato And Carrot Soup 75

Cooked Peas And Seitan 76

Bimi Cream 77

Broccoli And Almonds Cream 78

Pumpkin Cream 79

Chestnut Cream And Boniato 80

Carrot Mayonnaise 81

Avocado, Green Apple, Lime And Mint Cream 82

Mushroom Cream 83

Lombarda Cream 84

Potato Soup 85

Mushroom Cream Soup And Rice 86

Vegetable Soup 87

Zucchinis Soup 88

Stewed Tofu 89

Vegetable Stew 90

Basque Porrusalda 91

Chapter 3 92

Salads 92

Vegan Mushroom And Tofu 92

Quinoa Salad 94

Quinoa California Salad 95

Greek Pasta Salad 96

Thai Salad 97

Kale Salad With Chickpeas And Avocado 98

Chickpea Salad With Avocado 99

Lentil Salad 100

Perfect Summer Pasta Salad 101
Asparagus Salad With Blueberries And Vinaigrette 102
Kale Salad 103

Chapter 4 104

Pasta & Noodles 104

Vegan Noodles 104
Zucchini Pasta 105
Asian Spaghetti With Peanut Butter And Chilli 106
Pasta To Orange With Soybean 107
Pasta With Almond Cream, Red Pepper And Basil 108
Pasta To Pesto With Bimi 109
Pasta With Mushrooms And Tofu Sauce 110
Ramen 111
Noodles With Tofu And Peanut Dressing 112
Pasta With Vegan Pesto 114
Pasta With Avocado Cream 115
Pasta With Cheese Mix 116

Chapter 5 117

Rice & Grains 117

Granola, Greek Yogurt And Red Berries 117
Integral Rice With Pineapple And Coconut 118
Almond And Coconut Granola 119
Mango And Peach Smoothie Bowl 120
Organic Quinoa 121
Quinoa With Boricua Flavor 122
Instant Couscous 123
Rice, Beans And Kale With Dressing 124
Risotto Of Quinoa 125
Rice With Lentils 126
Choclo Grill 127
Chickpeas With Spinach 128
Rice With Vegetables 129

Integral Rice With Heura 130

Couscous With Vegetables 131

Sarraceno Wheat With Curry 132

Chapter 6 133

Vegetables 133

Baked Mushrooms 133

Fried Sweet Potato 134

Fried Cauliflowers 135

Baked Artichoke 136

Vegan Pancakes With Vegetables 137

Chocolate Oatmeal 138

Vegetarian Tacos 139

Mushroom Leek Quiche 140

Vegan Cheese Fingers 142

Escalivada 143

Green Beans With Tomato And Textured Soybean 144

Vegetable Tempura 145

Seitan With Peas Sauce 146

Tofu And Cereal Wraps 148

Asturian Vegan Tortos 149

Rustic Potatoes With Turmeric 150

Sweet And Sour Tofu With Peppers 151

Spicy Tofu With Honey And Sesame 152

Bimi Toast With Beet Hummus 153

Vegan Barbecue Pizza 154

Chickpea Pilaf 155

Vegan Potato and Cauliflower Quiche 156

Vegan Meatballs Of Brown Rice 157

Kentucky Fried Cauliflower 158

Flourless Spinach Pancakes 159

Vegan Ricotta 161

Aubergine Sandwich With Hummus 162

Vegan French Toast 163

Carrot Pancake 164

Revolted Tofu 165

Vegetarian Huarache..166

Portobello Stuffed With Quinoa..167

Barbecue Vegan Burritos 169

Oriental Style Vegetables 170

Jamaican Flower Tacos 171

Vegan Burrito In Bowl...172

Vegetable Stuffed Courgettes 174

Vegan Ceviche 176

Pico Of Gallo 177

Curled Lentils With Spinach 178

Peruvian Sautéed Loin 179

Chickpea And Avocado Sandwich 180

Mediterranean Nachos 181

Vegetarian Vegetable Lasagna 182

Vegetarian Pizza 184

Sweet Potatoes Stuffed With Black Beans 185

Chapter 6 186

Snacks & Sides 186

Tlacoyos Of Beans With Nopales Stew 186

Vegan & Gluten-Free Cookies Of Walnut And Blueberries..187

Vegan Sushi 188

Japanese Omelette Rice 189

Swiss-Style Potato And Onion Omelette 190

Potato, Ginger And Onion Tortilla...191

Lentil And Vegetable Burger 192

Zucchini Fritters 193

Roasted Cauliflower 194

Vegan Portobello Pizza 195

Peppers Stuffed With Quinoa And Vegetables 196

Grilled Pumpkin 197

Vegetarian Nuggets 198

Chapter 7 199
Desserts 199

- Baked Onion Rings 199
- Pasta Roll Stuffed with Spinach and Ricotta 200
- Potato Balls 201
- Vegetables And Tofu Skewers 202
- Fried Banana 203
- Chips Potatoes 204
- Caramelized Onion 205
- Watermelon Gazpacho 206
- Tofu And Chocolate Mousse 207
- Carrot Cake 208
- Carrot And Tofu Cake 210
- Strawberry Cream Cake 211
- Quince Sweet 212
- Oat And Banana Cookies 213
- Orange and Chocolate Cake 214
- Vegan Kefir 215
- Azteca Cake 216
- Strawberry Milkshake 217
- Potato and Mushroom Cake 218
- Oat Milk 219
- Strawberry Biscuit Cake 220
- Red Fruit Shake 221
- Oreo Crepes Tower 222
- Coriander And Walnut Pesto 223
- Hazelnut Milk With Cocoa 224
- Tofu Cream: Spreadable Tofu Cheese 225
- Almond Milk 226
- Ginger Milk 227
- Fresh Mint And Basil Ice Cream 228
- Watermelon Smoothie 229
- Banana Puccino 230

Vegan Potato Cheese 231

Purple smoothie 232

Coffee Truffles 233

Vegan Corn Cake 234

Vegan Cocoa Muffins 235

Vegan Chocolate Peanut Butter Cheesecake 236

Vegan Chocolate Pudding 237

21 Day meal plan for Plant-based Diet 238

Conclusion 242

Introduction

Plant-Based is a type of diet that, mainly, is based on consuming plants (understood as all vegetables, vegetables, legumes, cereals, etc.). That is, in reducing the consumption of products of animal origin.

It is a somewhat more flexible method than vegan or vegetarian because it does not eliminate animal consumption but it is considerably reduced. In this way, a healthier and greener diet is followed day by day and the environmental impact is reduced and, also, encourages

Plant-based, vegetarian, and vegan food can be super healthy and energetic in any cycle of life if it is done in a complete and varied way. Incorporate more real food into the daily diet. Add fresh vegetables and fruits, seeds, whole grains, legumes, nuts, algae, superfoods such as maca, spirulina, provide the body with quality food and all the nutrients necessary for proper functioning, purifying it, and recovering its self-healing capacity.

The key is to stop consuming so many packages, ultra-processed products with base ingredients such as wheat flour, corn, and soybeans, sugar, fats, full of chemicals, flavors, colors, that do not nourish and generate addiction. Everything vegan is not synonymous with healthy. Many vegan foods fall into these groups when eaten in excess, for example, seitan, soy, choriveganos, some commercial cookies, dressings, sodas, and more.

Do you remember the phrase, are you what you eat? As we are certainly much more than what we eat, the scientific evidence is showing more and more than what we eat affects us. Choosing the foods, we put on our plates — and which ones we avoid — gives us unprecedented power to live longer healthier lives.

Allowed food on a plant-based diet?

Although this name may seem to suggest that with this diet we can only eat plants, the truth is that it is something broader. It refers to eating a more vegetable diet and reducing the consumption of products of animal origin. Thus, within this new food method, the following foods can be consumed:

- Vegetables and greens
- Fruits
- Grain
- Walnuts
- Seeds
- Vegetables

And, yes, to get a healthy diet what you have to choose is to choose that these foods are as little processed as possible. In other words, the equation is simple: increase fruits and vegetables to the detriment of meat and fish, mainly.

The secret to the success of this type of diet is that it is a much healthier method for our body. But, also, it is a diet that is more respectful with the environment and that reduces our ecological impact. Also, the consumption of meat or fish from large-scale companies or factories that may keep animals in rather questionable health and living conditions is reduced.

By basing the highest amount of plant intakes, you transform your diet into a more alkaline and physiological one, incorporating food-medicine within its many benefits:

- Plants are high in fiber, which provides satiety, controls the absorption of glucose avoiding peaks of glycemia, stimulates the correct evacuation.
- They have antioxidants, prevent premature aging, have anti-cancer, and anti-inflammatory neuroprotective effects.
- They have a high concentration of vitamins and minerals: by consuming whole plants, a good dose of vitamins and minerals is provided, enzymatic cofactors of many metabolic reactions of the organism, which stimulates the general biochemical functionality of the body, increases energy, and improves the state of spirit.
- They are cleansing, they help eliminate toxins through our cleansing organs, liver, kidney, urine, fecal matter, perspiration.
- They alkalize the body, which helps to compensate for acidosis caused by excess consumption of meat and/or processed foods.
- It is important to accompany the transition to a plant-based diet, - vegan or vegetarian -with complete blood tests with vitamin B12 and homocysteine dosages, to assess the state of health and supplementation protocol, since it is not covered with foods of plant origin, it is very normal that in cases of flexible vegetarians without nutritional control, sometime after the change of diet, the values drop and symptoms appear.

Basic Ingredients and Shopping List

For some, it is very simple to make a Plant-Based shopping list, go to the supermarket, buy and organize the weekly menu. For others, it is the most difficult task they face every Sunday night. If the idea is also to start taking care of food and leading a healthy lifestyle, having a plan outlined seems to many an impossible mission.

Below, some points must be taken into account when going to the supermarket and how to combine them to lead a balanced lifestyle.

The 5 Basic Pillars of the Plant-Based Shopping List

1- Eat at least 3 pieces of fruit a day

The fruit is undoubtedly one of the foods that should not be missing in your cupboard. I generally buy apples, bananas, and some other seasonal fruit. Although it is not a fruit I do not want to forget about lemons and ginger.

Apples seem essential as they combine well with all foods. They can be used to prepare green smoothies, porridges, add them to a bowl of cereals and vegetable kinds of milk, or eat them alone during the day when hunger strikes. You can carry them in your bag to eat them as a snack.

Bananas are allies when it comes to preparing delicious vegan ice cream and satiating the desire for sweets. Remember to choose the ones with skin with brown spots since they are the sweetest. It is also the best time to ripen to consume them and thus take advantage of all their properties.

Seasonal fruits: The rest of the fruits you buy can be in season so you will ensure that they are fresh. In the winter oranges and tangerines are preferable. In the summer

Peaches, melons, plums, strawberries, watermelons, grapes, pylons, pineapples, etc. are great. This will of course depend on the country in which you live since in tropical climates we will find many more varieties.

With lemons, you can prepare your warm water with lemon and bicarbonate to drink every morning before breakfast.

Avocados: Although it has a slightly salty flavor, the avocado is considered a fruit. Never miss it in your shopping cart. Use it to spread my gluten-free bread to replace butter and cheese and to make a tasty vegan chocolate mousse.

Ginger is a root to include in this group. It is highly nutritious, anti-inflammatory, and antioxidant food. Use it every day in your green smoothies or salads.

2- Buy all kinds of vegetables

It is recommended to include in your shopping list Plant-Based a good assortment of vegetables so your dishes will be more creative and tastier. Below, an example of what is usually purchased:

- **Green leaves:** lettuce, arugula, Swiss chard, etc.
- Broccoli or cauliflower
- White or purple cabbage
- Carrots
- Zucchini or zucchini
- Onions
- Garlic
- Aubergines
- Tomatoes
- Cucumber
- Celery
- Artichokes
- Potatoes or potatoes
- Leeks

The idea is to combine raw and cooked vegetables with each meal. Although raw or live food is very fashionable now, not all people tolerate it as it is difficult for them to digest. The recommendation is that if it doesn't feel good to eat completely raw food, combine them on the same plate with cooked vegetables.

3- A good supply of carbohydrates, cereals, grains, and wholemeal flour

This group of foods is necessary for the correct functioning of the organism since they provide the necessary energy for the activities of daily life. The idea is to consume whole grains for their high fiber content that provides satiety and lowers its glycemic index.

- Choose 2 or 3 cereals per week and alternate each day to not always consume them. They can be quinoa and brown rice. You can also buy amaranth, rice or corn noodles, buckwheat, oats, etc. A quinoa and vegetable salad is ideal to eat at noon.
- You can choose the ones you prefer but try not to always consume the same cereal since each one provides different nutrients. Remember that it is best to consume them at noon so that you can "burn" them during the day.

- Within this group, bread is also included. Try to eat bread made with wholemeal flours that will give you more fiber and satiety with a lower glycemic index. You have several recipes on the blog for different combinations of gluten-free and wholemeal flours.

4- Legumes are the best source of vegetable protein?

- With legumes do the same as with cereals: Choose 2 different ones and consume them alternately during the week. They can be with lentils and chickpeas.
- With lentils, you can prepare hamburgers, include them in salads or make delicious stews.
- Chickpeas also allow various preparations such as hummus to accompany salads, raw vegetables or spread bread, make vegan burgers, falafel, include them in salads, or prepare stews.
- Other legumes that you can consume are the azuki or adukis, the beans or black beans, the beans, etc.

5- Includes nuts and seeds

Although they are last on the list, it is considered an extremely important group for its contribution of proteins, fats, and essential nutrients.

- As for the seeds, the indispensable ones are sesame seeds, chia seeds, and flax seeds. Sesame seeds are used to prepare the vegetable milk you consume daily due to their high calcium content.
- Chia and flax seeds are used to add to green smoothies or cereal and fruit bowls. They are highly antioxidant, anti-inflammatory, and have a high percentage of vitamins and minerals.
- Choose nuts such as almonds, hazelnuts, cashews (cashews), and walnuts. Being a group of foods with a high price you can choose one of them and consume a handful every day along with a piece of fruit, for example, add them to a green smoothie or use them to prepare vegetable milk.

Other Foods To Complete Your Plant-Based Shopping List

- Usually eat chocolate, grated coconut, raisins, dates, coconut oil, natural sweeteners, and tahini (sesame paste).
- Raisins and dates, as mentioned before, are used to prepare truffles or to eat them alone when you need a share of sweets.
- Coconut oil is used to spread gluten-free bread to replace butter.
- As for natural sweeteners, it is good to use stevia leaves, but if you cannot do without them, it is advisable to use agave and rice syrups, coconut sugar, or Muscovy sugar.
- Finally, tahin is another food that is used to spread bread. It is bought ready or you can do it yourself by processing roasted sesame seeds until their oil begins to spread and they transform into pasta or butter.
- Condiments and spices: spices cannot be missing from your cupboard to enhance the flavor of your meals: oregano, turmeric, curry, pepper, dill, garlic powder, paprika, and salt is also very important. Remember to buy Himalayan salt or another salt that is not refined.

Chapter 1

Breakfast

Avocado Toast

Servings: 2-4
Preparation time: 5 minutes
Cook time: 5 minutes

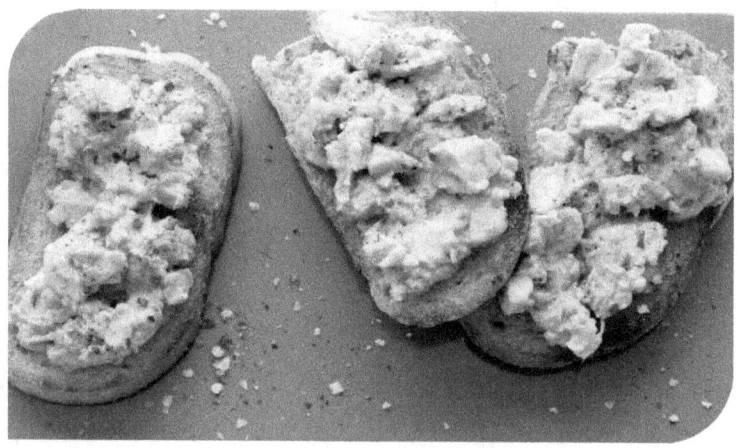

Ingredients

- 4 slices of whole wheat bread
- 1 avocado, cut in half and pitted
- 1 tablespoon of lemon juice
- ½ teaspoon garlic powder
- Pinch of sea salt

Steps to Cook

1. Toast the bread in a toaster or toaster oven.
2. While the bread is toasting, place the avocado in a bowl.
3. 3 Add the lemon juice, garlic powder and salt, and mash with a fork or potato masher.
4. 4 Trim the nori leaf or dark lettuce and ready to eat.

Nutritional Information:

- Calorie: 620
- Protein: 23g
- Fat: 42g
- Carbohydrates: 48g

Vegan Pancakes

Servings: 2
Preparation time: 5 minutes
Cook time: 5 minutes

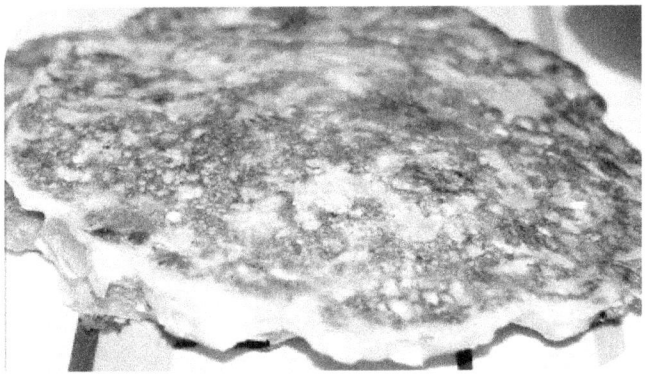

Ingredients

For the pancakes
- ½ cup chickpea flour
- ½ cup of water

For filling:
- 1 large zuchini
- 2 carrots
- 1 onion
- Garlic
- Salt
- Turmeric
- Pepper
- Coconut milk or other vegetable cream

Steps to Cook

1. Place the chickpea flour and water in a deep bowl and beat to integrate well with an electric or wire whisk.
2. Heat over medium-low heat in a medium nonstick skillet to cook pancakes. Add a few drops of oil to prevent the dough from sticking. Once the pan is very hot, add a few tablespoons of the preparation to make the first pancake. Once the edges begin to peel off, turn it over to cook on the other side. Repeat the process two more times. Reserve the pancakes.

For the filling:
3. Chop the onion and cook it in a pan with oil until it becomes transparent. Meanwhile, peel and cut the carrot and zuchini into cubes of the desired size. Also chop the garlic. Pour the garlic, carrot and zuchini into the pan and cook for a few minutes until the vegetables are tender. Finally add turmeric, pepper and serve.

Nutritional Information:

- Calorie: 73.9
- Protein: 3g
- Fat: 0.3g
- Carbohydrates: 15.8g

Chocolate Oatmeal

Servings: 2
Preparation time: 5 minutes
Cook time: 5 minutes

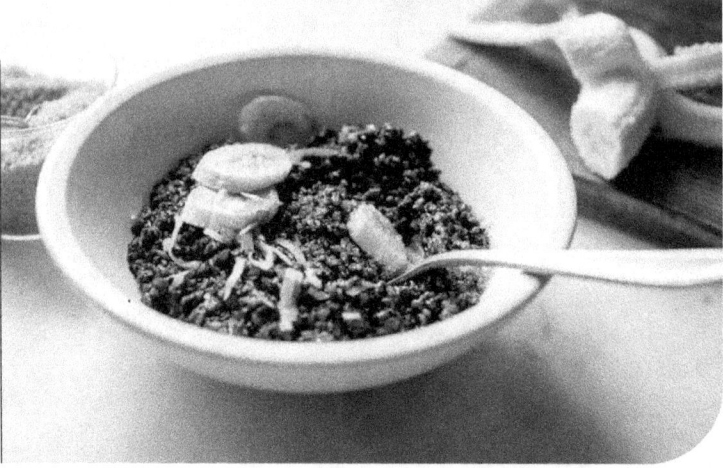

Ingredients

- 2 cups divided unsweetened plant-based milk
- 5-6 seedless dates
- ¾ cup oat flakes
- 1 ½ tablespoon cocoa powder
- ½ teaspoon cinnamon
- 1 tablespoon chia seeds
- Fresh or thawed strawberries or cherries

Steps to Cook

1. Combine one cup of the almond milk with the dates in a blender until the dried fruits are crushed well and the consistency is creamy.
2. Transfer the mixture along with the additional cup of milk to a medium saucepan and add the rest of the ingredients except the fruits.
3. Bring to a simmer and cook over medium heat until thickened, about 15 minutes.
4. Add additional milk if the oatmeal is too thick for your taste.
5. Serve with bananas.

Nutritional Information:

- Calorie: 160
- Protein: 6g
- Fat: 3g
- Carbohydrates: 30g

Vegetarian Tacos

Servings: 4
Preparation time: 5 minutes
Cook time: 5 minutes

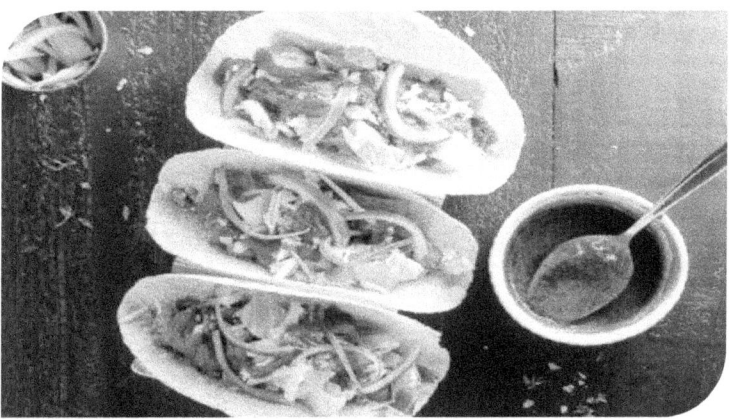

Ingredients

- 1 tbsp of vegetable oil
- ½ cup red onion
- ½ cups green or red bell pepper
- 15.25 oz black beans unsalted
- 15.25 oz. corn kernels, unsalted
- 1 teaspoon of ground cumin
- 2 cups of water
- 1 package Taco Rice
- 2 tablespoons fresh coriander

Steps to Cook

1. Heat oil in large nonstick skillet over medium-high heat and cook onion, bell pepper, beans, corn, and cumin, stirring occasionally, for about 5 minutes. Stir and reserve.
2. Add the water and Taco Rice in the same pan and bring to a boil. Reduce heat to low and simmer, covered, for 7 minutes or until rice is tender.
3. Incorporate the vegetables; Let stand covered for 2 minutes. Add the coriander. If desired, serve with your favorite taco side dishes, such as diced avocado, tomato, onion, grated cheese, lime wedges, sour cream, sliced radishes, and hot sauce; now they are delicious. Enjoy it!

Nutritional Information:

- Calorie: 407
- Protein: 19.7g
- Fat: 6.4g
- Carbohydrates: 74.4g

Instant Oats

Servings: 2-4
Preparation time: 5 minutes
Cook time: 5 minutes

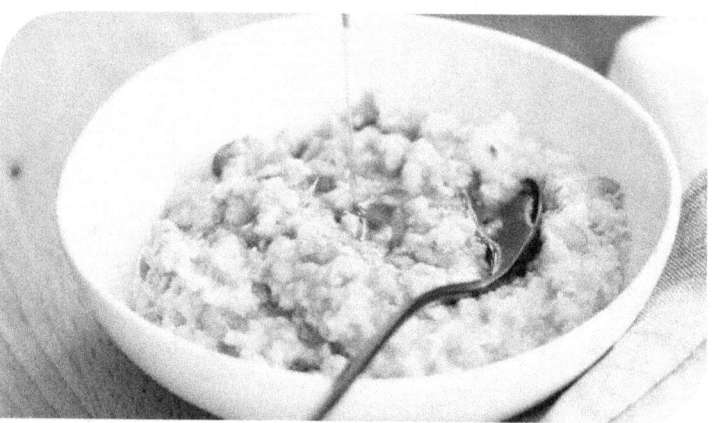

Ingredients

- ½ cup oatmeal
- ½ – ⅔ cup hot or cold water
- ½ cup of vegetable milk
- 1 teaspoon of maqui berry powder
- ½ cup fresh grapes or berries
- Half banana
- Walnuts
- Seeds

Steps to Cook

1. Combine the oatmeal and water in a bowl, and let them soak for a few minutes.
2. Cut the banana and the grapes or berries as desired, and add them to the oats.
3. Pour the vegetable milk over the oats and fruits.
4. Top with nuts, seeds, powdered maqui berry, or acai powder. You can use walnut nuts and hemp seeds.

Nutritional Information:

- Calorie: 389
- Protein: 16.9g
- Fat: 6.9g
- Carbohydrates: 66.3g

Vegan Bread

Servings: 2-4
Preparation time: 25 minutes
Cook time: 45 minutes

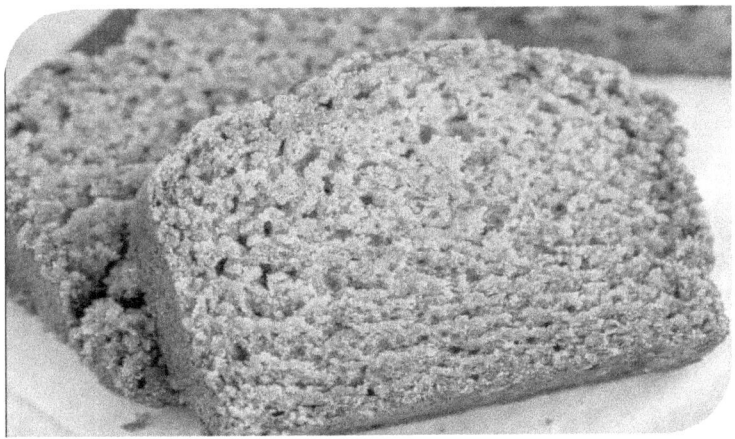

Ingredients

- ½ lbs. coral lentils
- ¼ lbs. of millet
- 1 tablespoon of vinegar or lemon
- 1 teaspoon salt
- Water
- Spices to taste (turmeric, ginger, pepper, etc.)

Steps to Cook

1. Place the lentils and millet in a bowl. Cover them with water and let stand 12 hours. After that time, rinse the grains, discarding the soaking water.
2. Crush the lentils and millet with a minipimer or food processor to form a sticky dough. Add the vinegar or the lemon, the salt and the chosen spices and mix.
3. Let the dough rest in a bowl covered with plastic wrap or with a kitchen cloth at room temperature for two days. After that time, the dough begins to rise and you will feel an acidic smell due to the fermentation of the grains. Place the dough in a previously oiled bread pan or upholstered with vegetable paper.
4. Take in a preheated oven at 180 ° about 30-40 minutes or until a toothpick is inserted and it comes out dry.

Nutritional Information:

- Calorie: 80
- Protein: 1g
- Fat: 2g
- Carbohydrates: 14g

Sweet Potatoes Toast And Blueberries

Servings: 2
Preparation time: 5 minutes
Cook time: 20 minutes

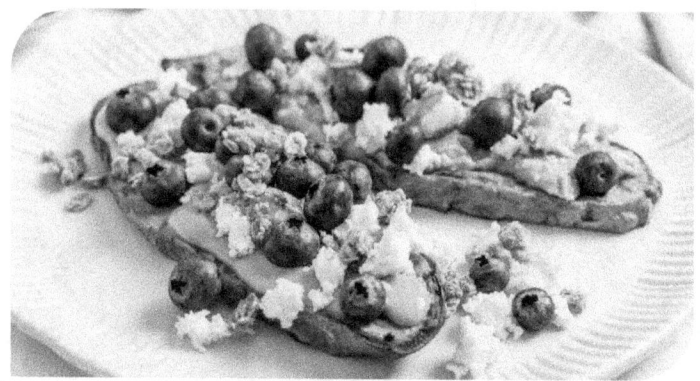

Ingredients

- 1 sweet potato, cut into slices half a centimeter thick
- ¼ cup almond butter
- ½ cup blueberries

Steps to Cook

1. Preheat oven to 240°F.
2. Place the sweet potato slices on baking paper. Bake until smooth, about 20 minutes. (You can also cook them in a toaster, but you would need to turn it on high for three to four cycles.)
3. Serve hot, top with peanut butter and blueberries. Store any leftover sweet potato slices, without dressing, in an airtight container in the refrigerator for a week. Reheat them in a toaster or toaster oven and cover as directed.

Nutritional Information:

- Calorie: 170
- Protein: 3g
- Fat: 9g
- Carbohydrates: 21g

Pasta With Lemon, Asparagus And Cauliflower

Servings: 2-4
Preparation time: 5 minutes
Cook time: 20 minutes

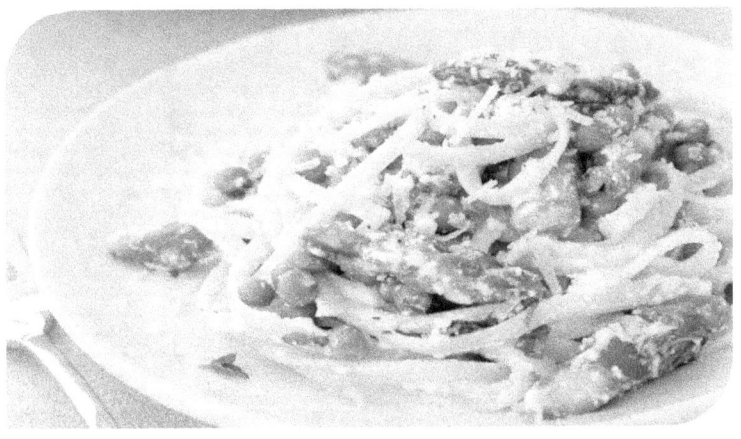

Ingredients

- 2 tbsp olive oil, divided
- 3 cups of various colored cauliflower sprigs
- 2 cups of water, divided
- ¼ cup 2% milk
- 1 package of Lemon & Asparagus with Cavatappi spaghetti
- 1 cup cannellini beans, canned, washed
- ¼ cup low-fat ricotta cheese
- ¼ cup chopped and toasted walnuts

Steps to Cook

1. Heat 1 tablespoon of olive oil in a large nonstick skillet over medium-high heat and cook the cauliflower, stirring occasionally, until golden, about 5 minutes. Add ½ cup water to the skillet and cook 5 minutes or until cauliflower is tender. Remove the cauliflower and set aside.
2. Pour the remaining 1 ½ cups of water, milk, and the remaining tablespoon of olive oil in the same pan. Bring to a boil. Stir the package of spaghetti and bring to a boil, then lower heat to medium-high and simmer for 8 minutes, covered and stirring frequently.
3. Add the cauliflower and beans. Add ricotta to center. Garnish with walnuts and, if desired, with fresh parsley or chopped basil. Now it was delicious, try it!

Nutritional Information:

- Calorie: 489
- Protein: 13g
- Fat: 4g
- Carbohydrates: 96g

Zucchini Rolls Stuffed With Dried Tomato Paté

Servings: 2-4
Preparation time: 10 minutes
Cook time: 10 minutes

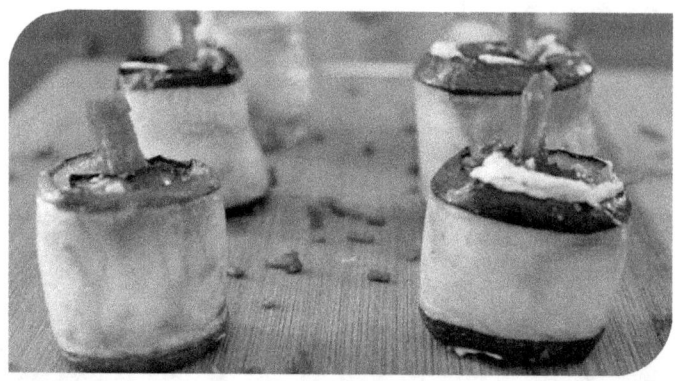

Ingredients

- 1 zucchini
- ½ cup cashews or cashews
- 8 dried tomatoes
- Fresh basil leaves
- A few drops of lemon
- 1 tablespoon of olive oil
- Salt and pepper to taste

Steps to Cook

1. Wash the zuchini well. Using a mandolin or a knife, cut it into very thin sheets. Arrange them on a plate and add salt so that they soften a little so that they can be rolled up more easily.
2. To prepare the filling, place the dried tomatoes in a bowl, add boiling water to hydrate them and let them rest for about 10 minutes.
3. Place the cashews in the glass of the blender or food processor. Add salt, a few drops of lemon, a tablespoon of olive oil, fresh basil and the hydrated tomatoes. Process until all the ingredients are well integrated and obtain a homogeneous paste.
4. To finish, arrange a sheet of zuchini on a plate, spread it with a teaspoon of dried tomato paté and roll it up.

Nutritional Information:

- Calorie: 489
- Protein: 13g
- Fat: 4g
- Carbohydrates: 96g

Vegetable Seasoned Oats

Servings: 4-6
Preparation time: 10 minutes
Cook time: 7-10 minutes

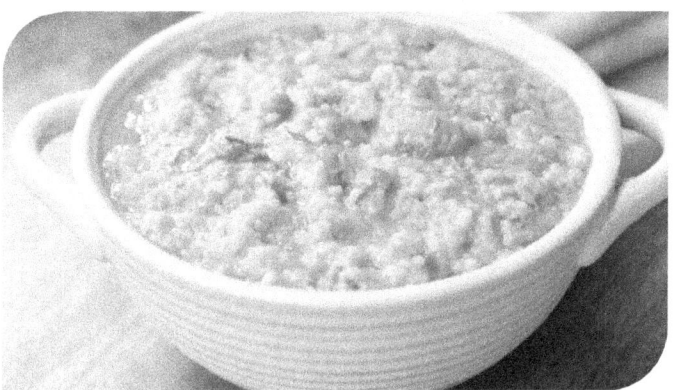

Ingredients

- 2 cups of "cut" oats
- ½ teaspoon sea salt
- 1 teaspoon Italian spices
- 1 tsp garlic powder
- 4 cups of water
- ½ cup nutritional yeast
- 1 teaspoon onion powder
- ¼ tsp turmeric powder
- ½ cup mushrooms
- ¼ cup grated carrots
- 1 ½ cup kale or tender spinach
- ½ cup small peppers

Steps to Cook

1. Boil the water in a saucepan.
2. Add the oats and spices and lower the temperature.
3. Cook over low heat without lid for 5 to 7 minutes.
4. Add the vegetables.
5. Cover and set aside for 2 minutes.
6. Serve immediately.

Nutritional Information:

- Calorie: 90
- Protein: 2.4g
- Fat: 3.3g
- Carbohydrates: 12.7g

Vegan Pea Burger

Servings: 12
Preparation time: 20 minutes
Cook time: 35 minutes

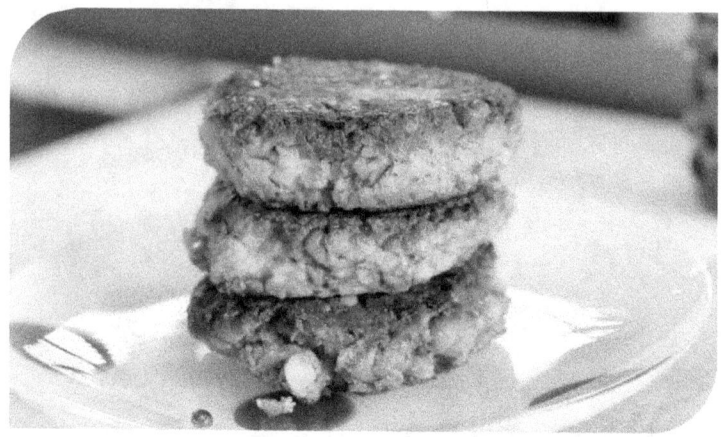

Ingredients

- 2 cups cooked peas
- 1 cup of oatmeal
- 1 cooked carrot
- ½ cup black olives
- Garlic
- Salt and spices to taste

Steps to Cook

1. Put the oats in a mixer and process it into a thick flour (you can also use the whole flakes if you prefer)
2. On the other hand, pour the peas or peas, the carrot, the olives and the garlic in the glass of a food processor or minipimer. Crush well to a sticky mass.
3. Place the preparation in a bowl and add the desired salt and spices. Mix well.
4. Finally add the oats to give a more compact consistency to the dough. Integrate well.
5. Take portions of dough by hand and form hamburgers of the desired size.
6. Arrange them on a previously oiled baking sheet. Cook in a preheated oven at 180 °C for about 15 minutes on each side or until the surface of the patties is golden

Nutritional Information:

- Calorie: 167
- Protein: 21.3g
- Fat: 4.1g
- Carbohydrates: 11g

Vegan Tart

Servings: 8
Preparation time: 20 minutes
Cook time: 20 minutes

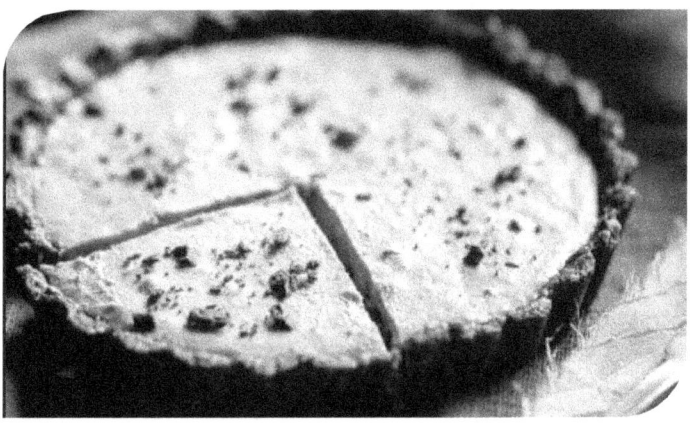

Ingredients

For the mass:
- ½ lbs. whole wheat flour
- 4 tablespoons of oil
- 2 cups of water
- 1 pinch of salt

For the filling:
- 2 leeks
- 2 cups of mushrooms
- 2 small onion
- 1 clove garlic
- 6 cherry tomatoes
- Salt, pepper and spices to taste
- 6 tbsp of chickpea flour
- 18 tablespoons of water
- 1 teaspoon of vinegar

Steps to Cook

For the mass:
1. In a bowl place the flour, oil, water and salt and mix well to form smooth dough.
2. Roll it out on a previously oiled cake pan or upholstered with vegetable paper. Pinch the dough with a fork.
3. Bake at 180°C for 10 minutes until slightly cooked.

For the filling:
4. In a frying pan, sauté the onions, leeks and garlic in olive oil. Add the mushrooms, salt, pepper and spices and sauté for a few more minutes.
5. Once it is well cooked, pour into a bowl and let it cool down a bit.
6. In another bowl place the chickpea flour, vinegar and water and form an egg-like cream.
7. Add this mixture to the vegetables and mix well.
8. Pour it over the previously cooked dough, decorate with cherrys cut in half and take to the oven for 10-15 more minutes until the edges of the dough are well cooked and the mixture of chickpea flour, vinegar and water has linked the ingredients.

Nutritional Information:

- Calorie: 278
- Protein: 4.4g
- Fat: 16.7g
- Carbohydrates: 28.9g

Oatmeal With Chia Seeds

Servings: 1
Preparation time: 2h

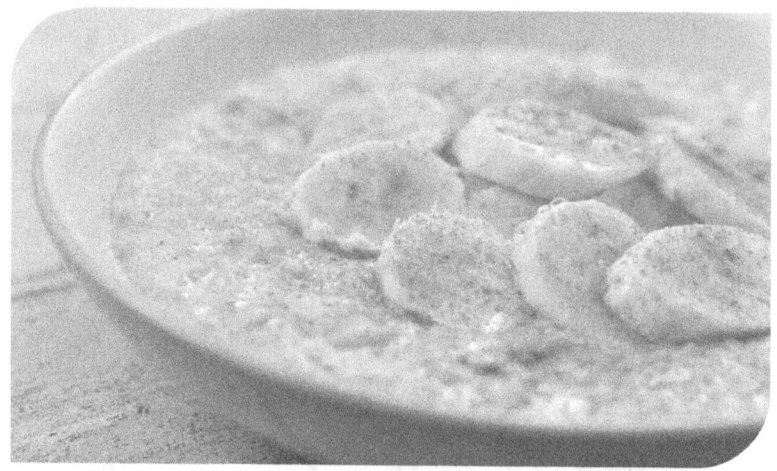

Ingredients

- 1.7 oz oats
- ¼ cup milk of your choice
- 2 tbsp chia seeds

Steps to Cook

1. Firstly, once you have your ingredients ready, in a bowl or glass add the oats, the chia seeds and finally the milk until it completely covers the container.
2. Mix the ingredients well.
3. Refrigerate for at least 2 hours so that the oats and chia absorb the milk and soften.
4. After 2 hours, add a little more milk so that it moistens more and the mixture does not dry out.

Nutritional Information:

- Calorie: 353.8
- Protein: 15.6g
- Fat: 8g
- Carbohydrates: 55.3g

Peanut Butter Pancakes

Servings: 4
Preparation time: 10 minutes
Cook time: 15 minutes

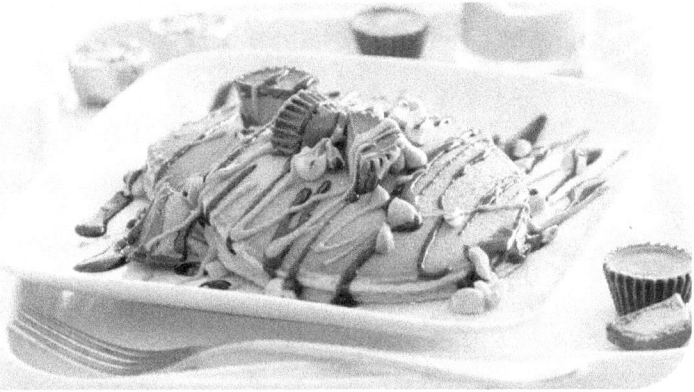

Ingredients

- 1 Cup of multipurpose flour
- 1 tsp baking powder
- ½ tsp baking soda
- ¼ tsp of salt
- ½ tsp ground cinnamon
- 1 egg
- 2 tablespoons of cream sugar
- 1 Tbsp of peanut butter
- 1 tsp vanilla extract
- 1 cup milk
- 1 tbsp butter
- 3 ripe bananas on wheels
- 1 cup of honey

Steps to Cook

1. Mix the multipurpose flour with the baking powder, the baking soda, the salt and the cinnamon in a bowl.
2. In another container, combine the egg, sugar, peanut butter, vanilla extract, and milk. Incorporate this mixture into the dry ingredients and combine well.
3. Meanwhile, heat the nonstick skillet or grill. Drizzle with oil spray or spread a little butter if you feel like it. Add about a quarter cup serving and cook on one side until bubbles start on one side, turn and cook thoroughly on the other side.
4. Serve with sliced bananas and honey.

Nutritional Information:

- Calorie: 140.6
- Protein: 5.2g
- Fat: 6.4g
- Carbohydrates: 17g

Vegetable Quiche

Servings: 4-6
Preparation time: 10 minutes
Cook time: 45-50 minutes

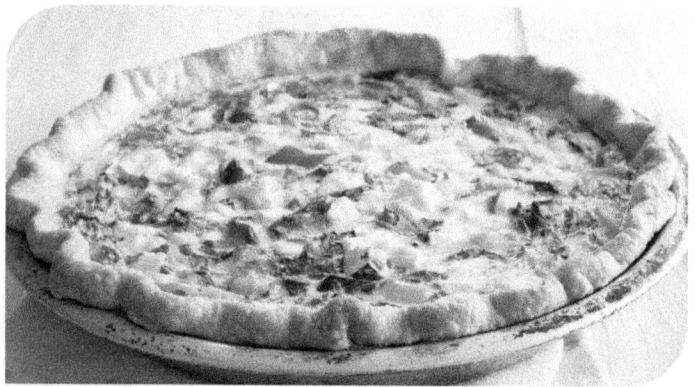

Ingredients

- Red cabbage
- White cabbage
- Onion
- Carrot
- Zucchini
- 2-3 eggs
- Liquid cream
- Salt
- cheese
- Puff pastry
- Tomatoes

Steps to Cook

1. Grate all the vegetables except the tomato and mix with the eggs and the cream. You add cream depending on the texture there should not be a liquid texture, rather solid, all compact.
2. Next, add the cheese and mix again.
3. Use a corrugated mold with a removable base, but put baking paper to extract the quiche once done. Spread the dough in it and prick several times with a fork. Bake the base at 180°C for 15 minutes.
4. Extract the base and fill with the mixture. Cover with a layer of cheese and tomatoes. Put a little oregano on top to give it more taste.
5. Bake the set for 30-35 minutes at 180°C. Until the filling is curdled and the golden mass. It is served hot and ready!

Nutritional Information:

- Calorie: 257
- Protein: 6g
- Fat: 17g
- Carbohydrates: 17g

Black Bean Flutes

Servings: 10
Preparation time: 5 minutes
Cook time: 5 minutes

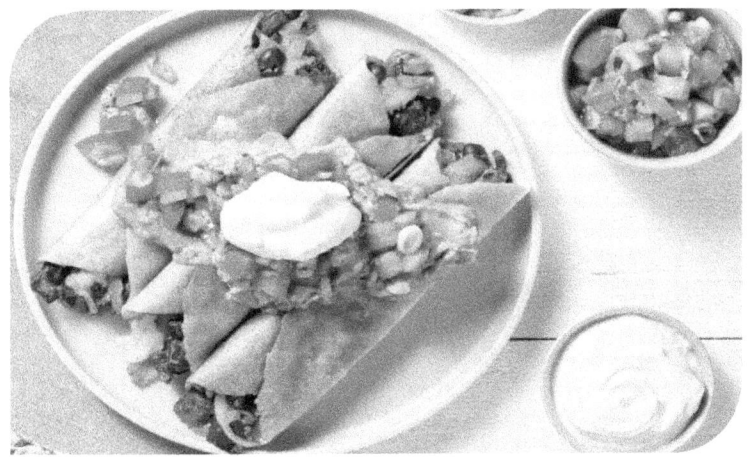

Ingredients

- 2 ½ cups cooked beans
- ½ chopped onion
- 2/3 cup Black Bean Broth
- 2 Chiles without seeds and chopped
- 1 tablespoon oil
- 12 corn tortillas
- ½ cup cream
- 1 cup cheese grated
- ¼ julienne romaine lettuce
- 2 cups red sauce oil to taste
- Salt, Pepper to taste

Steps to Cook

1. Season the onion and add the chilies.
2. Cook for 5 minutes.
3. Add the beans, the broth and the epazote.
4. Crush and pepper.
5. Cook until thick and dry. Remove and let cool.
6. Heat the tortillas and fill with the previous mixture.
7. Roll up to form flutes.
8. Fry until golden brown and drain on absorbent paper.
9. Serve and add the cream, lettuce and cheese and serve with the red sauce.

Nutritional Information:

- Calorie: 301.9
- Protein: 14g
- Fat: 4.3g
- Carbohydrates: 55.4g

Soy Milk And Oatmeal Smoothie

Servings: 1
Preparation time: 5 minutes

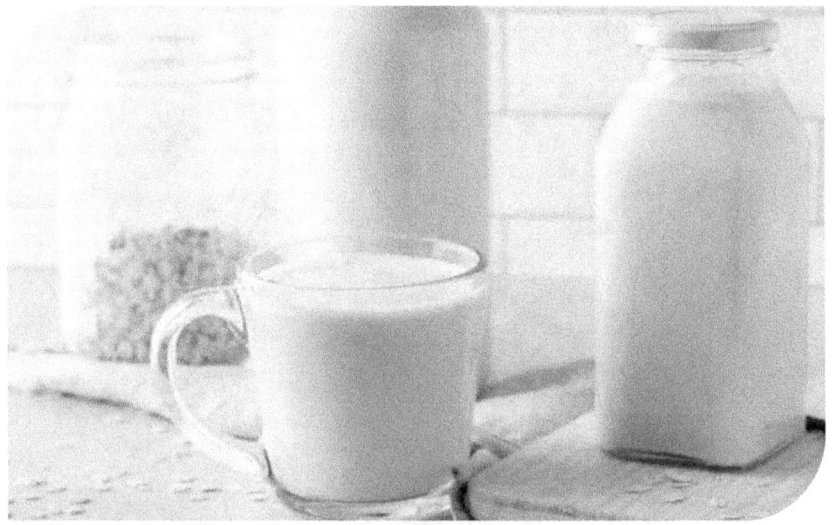

Ingredients

- ½ cup quick oatmeal
- 1 cup soy milk
- ½ cup of ice
- Sweetener to taste

Steps to Cook

1. Add all the ingredients to the blender for 5 minutes. It should be smooth.

Nutritional Information:

- Calorie: 120
- Protein: 3g
- Fat: 5g
- Carbohydrates: 16g

Vegan Omelette

Servings: 1
Preparation time: 5 minutes
Cook time: 5 minutes

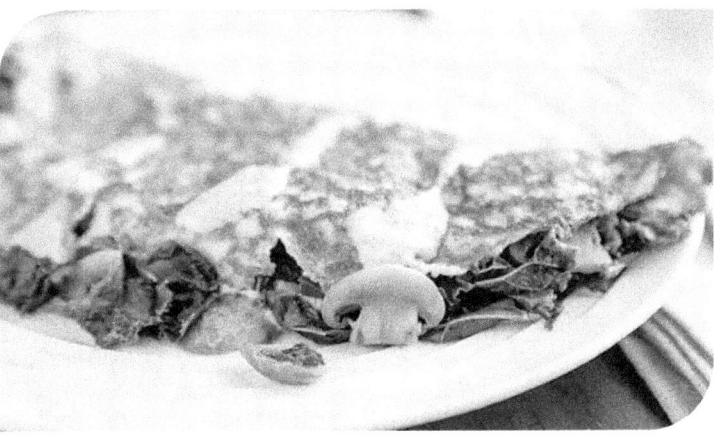

Ingredients

- 6 ounces Mori-nu lite silken tofu
- Cherry tomatoes
- Basil
- Olive oil
- cheese
- Salt and pepper

Steps to Cook

1. On a frying pan heat a teaspoon of olive oil and add 6 ounces Mori-nu lite silken tofu.
2. Now add the tomatoes, cheese, and basil.
3. Form a kind of omelette and roll.

Nutritional Information:

- Calorie: 104.5
- Protein: 11.3g
- Fat: 1.9g
- Carbohydrates: 10.2g

Pecan Butter

Servings: 4
Preparation time: 15 minutes
Cook time: 10 minutes

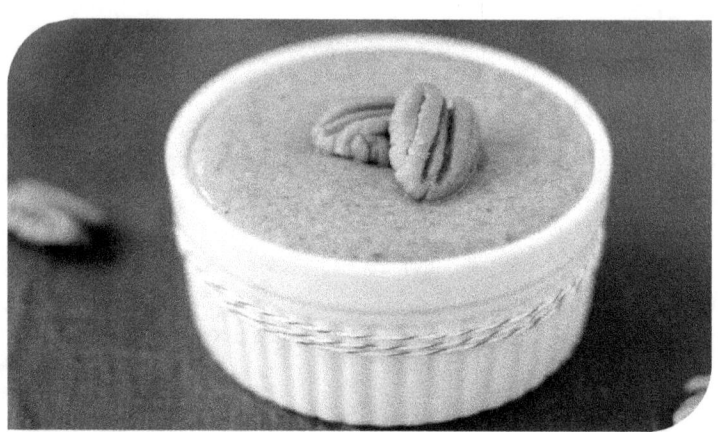

Ingredients

- 2 cups of raw walnuts of any kind
- Salt to taste
- Grape or canola seed oil, as needed (1 tbsp)

Steps to Cook

1. Preheat oven to 160 degrees.
2. Spread the walnuts on a rimmed baking sheet. Toast for 20 to 25 minutes, until they are toasted. Let cool for 2 to 3 minutes on the tray.
3. Add to food processor while hot and process 4 to 12 minutes until creamy, scraping down sides as needed (exact timing depends on your food processor). If the nuts are very dry and crumbly within a few minutes, add a tablespoon of oil during processing.
4. When creamy, add salt to taste (add ¼ tsp.).
5. Transfer walnut butter to a jar and keep refrigerated for up to 4 weeks.

Nutritional Information:

- Calorie: 170
- Protein: 2g
- Fat: 18g
- Carbohydrates: 4g

Rice Cakes

Servings: 4-6
Preparation time: 15 minutes
Cook time: 10 minutes

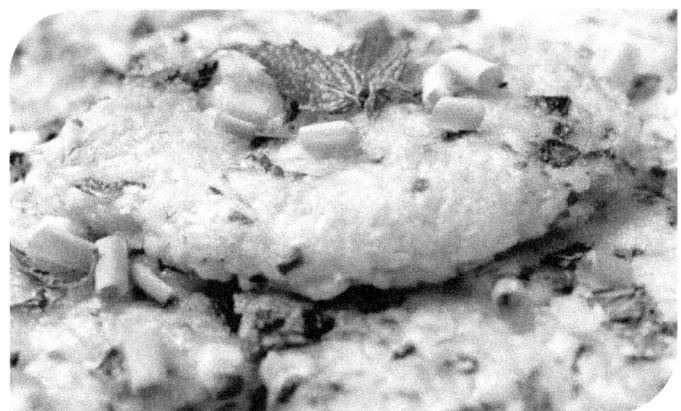

Ingredients

- 3 cups of preferably brown rice
- 1 cup of water or vegetable milk
- One tablespoon of olive oil.

to rectify flavors:

- Spices, herbs to taste.

Steps to Cook

1. Previously heat a non-stick frying pan well.
2. Blend the rice with the liquid and the other ingredients, it should be thick.
3. With a spoon we put a little of the dough in the pan and shape. They are not too thick but not so thin that they look like an omelette.
4. Cover and brown on both sides over medium heat.
5. Serve accompanied by a salty or sweet vegan sauce.
6. Remember that the rice is already cooked so it is only necessary to brown well on both sides.

Nutritional Information:

- Calorie: 35
- Protein: 0.7g
- Fat: 0.3g
- Carbohydrates: 7.3g

Oatmeal Pancakes

Servings: 4-6
Preparation time: 30 minutes
Cook time: 10-15 minutes

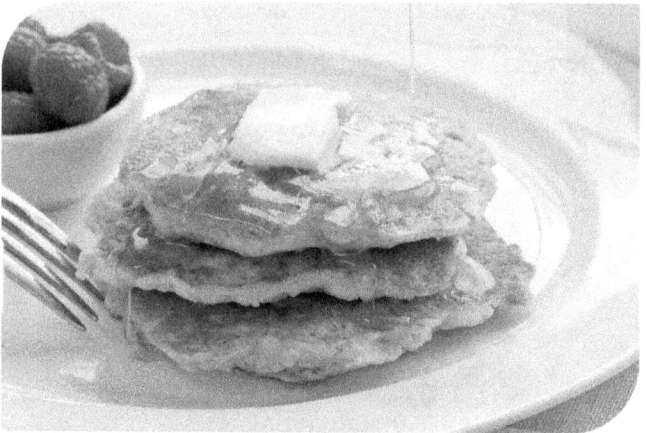

Ingredients

- 1 cup oatmeal
- Water with
- Pinch of salt
- ¾ cup grated coconut
- 1 shoreline baking powder
- 1 tbsp vinegar

optional:
- a banana (sweet) or grated carrot (salty)

Steps to Cook

1. Blend the cup of oatmeal with ½ cup of filtered water.
2. Add the rest of the ingredients minus the coconut.
3. Add more water until you get consistent dough like pancakes.
4. Add the grated coconut, stir well and let stand ½ hour in the fridge.
5. Heat a frying pan, cook the pancakes round and round and enjoy the topping you want.

Nutritional Information:

- Calorie: 159
- Protein: 4.9g
- Fat: 7.4g
- Carbohydrates: 18g

Chia Vegan Pancakes

Servings: 1
Preparation time: 15 minutes
Cook time: 10 minutes

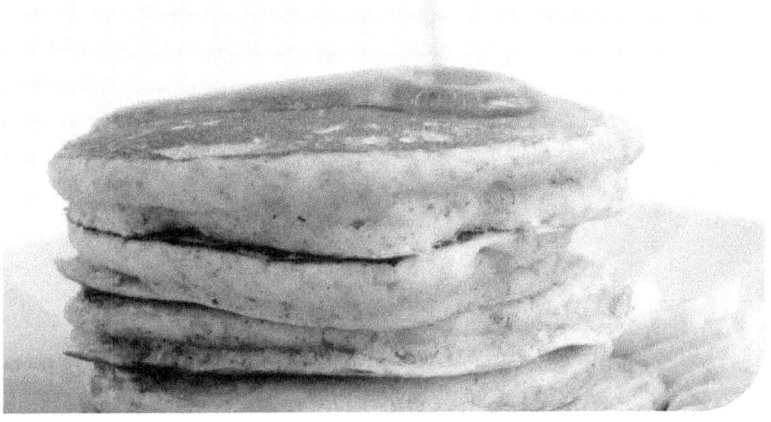

Ingredients

- 40 g oatmeal (if you don't have flour, grind the oatmeal)
- 1 tbsp chia seeds
- 1 tbsp sesame

Steps to Cook

1. Mix all the ingredients (except the oil) until creating a homogeneous paste (it should be a little liquid but not like water).
2. Let stand about 15 minutes minimum (so that the chia seeds are hydrated).
3. It can also be done at night and left to rest in the fridge overnight.
4. In a frying pan, add a little extra virgin olive oil or coconut oil and add a ladle of dough. we leave 23 minutes and turn.
5. Repeat until we finish with the dough.
6. Accompany fruit, nuts, grated coconut, cinnamon, natural soy yogurt, pure cocoa powder.

Nutritional Information:

- Calorie: 229.9
- Protein: 10.2g
- Fat: 6.9g
- Carbohydrates: 32.5g

Oatmeal Porridge

Servings: 1
Preparation time: 5 minutes
Cook time: 5 minutes

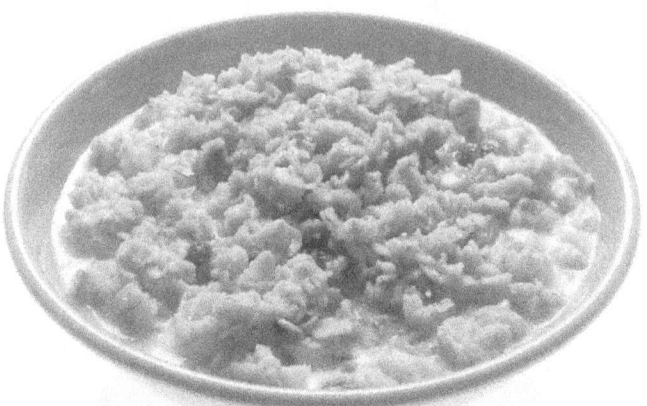

Ingredients

- 1 cup of oatmeal
- 2 cups of almond milk
- 1 teaspoon of peanut butter
- 1 banana
- Cinnamon
- Agave syrup

Steps to Cook

1. In a saucepan, boil the oatmeal with the milk and cinnamon until the oats soften and we have a slightly thick mixture.
2. Pour the mixture into a bowl and put banana, peanut butter and syrup on top.

Nutritional Information:

- Calorie: 214
- Protein: 11g
- Fat: 5.8g
- Carbohydrates: 30g

Chia Banana Porridge

Servings: 1
Preparation time: 10 minutes
Cook time: 15 minutes

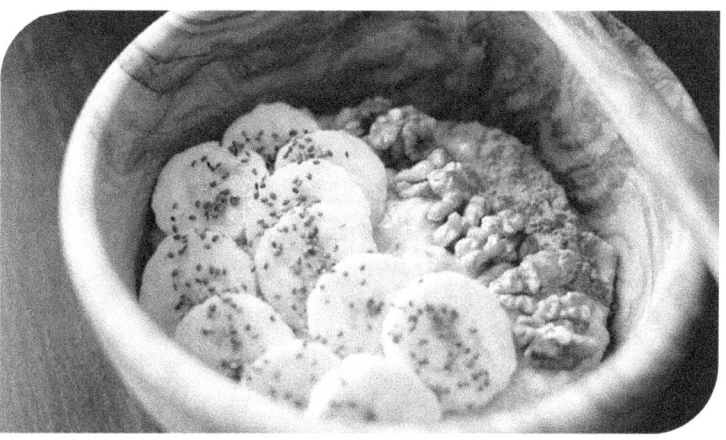

Ingredients

- 1 cup of oatmeal
- 2 cups of almond milk
- 1 teaspoon of peanut butter
- 1 banana
- Cinnamon
- Agave syrup

Steps to Cook

3. In a saucepan, boil the oatmeal with the milk and cinnamon until the oats soften and we have a slightly thick mixture.
4. Pour the mixture into a bowl and put banana, peanut butter and syrup on top.

Nutritional Information:

- Calorie: 214
- Protein: 11g
- Fat: 5.8g
- Carbohydrates: 30g

Blueberry Buckwheat Pancakes

Servings: 4
Preparation time: 10 minutes
Cook time: 25 minutes

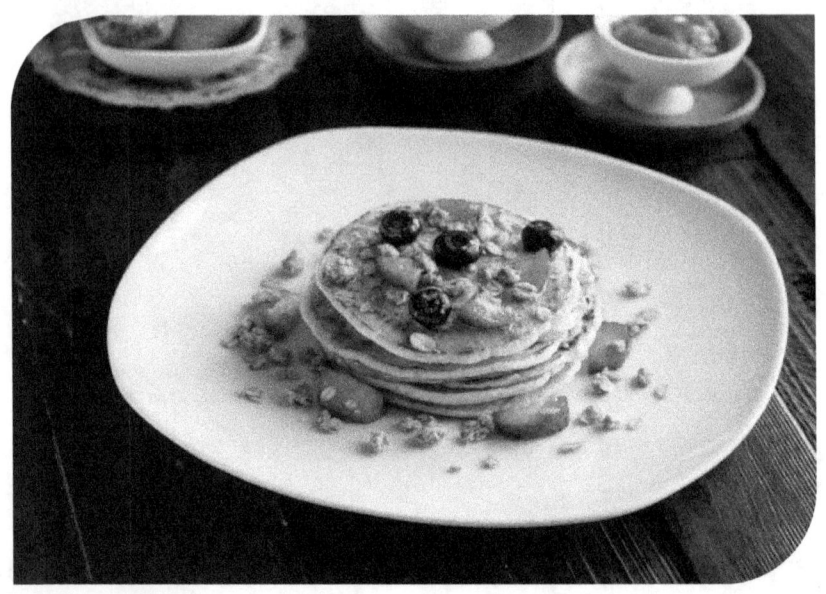

Ingredients

- ¼ cup chia seeds
- 1 tsp of green powder (optional)
- 2 tbsp fresh berries
- 1 tsp of cinnamon
- ½ to 1 ripe banana, mashed
- 1 tbsp coconut softened oil or nut butter

Steps to Cook

1. Stir in the soaked chia seeds until gelatinous consistency forms.
2. Add a little more liquid if desired. Add the banana puree.
3. Combine until the mixture has a consistency like porridge. Add cinnamon, green powder (if desired), coconut oil or pecan butter, and berries.
4. Serve in a deep plate and enjoy. Top with coconut flakes for added crunch.

Nutritional Information:

- Calorie: 91.4
- Protein: 3.7g
- Fat: 3.7g
- Carbohydrates: 11.9g

Oatmeal Soaks With Goji Berries

Servings: 1-2
Preparation time: 10 minutes
Cook time: 2-10 minutes

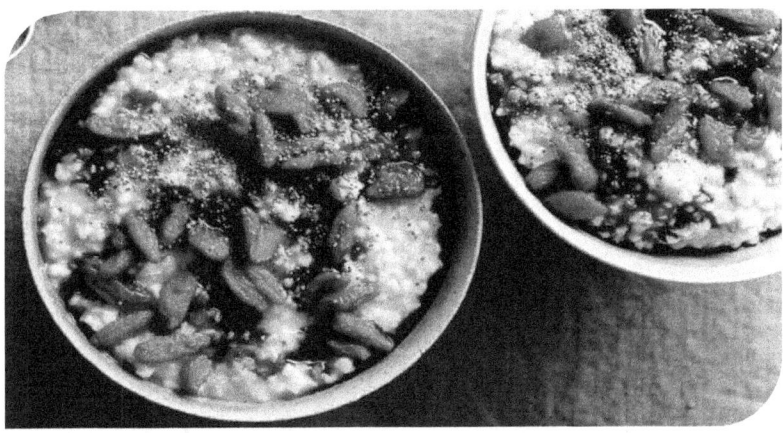

Ingredients

- ¼ cup chia seeds
- 1 tsp of green powder (optional)
- 2 tbsp fresh berries
- 1 tsp of cinnamon
- ½ to 1 ripe banana, mashed
- 1 tbsp coconut softened oil or nut butter

Steps to Cook

1. Stir in the soaked chia seeds until gelatinous consistency forms.
2. Add a little more liquid if desired. Add the banana puree.
3. Combine until the mixture has a consistency like porridge. Add cinnamon, green powder (if desired), coconut oil or pecan butter, and berries.
4. Serve in a deep plate and enjoy. Top with coconut flakes for added crunch.

Nutritional Information:

- Calorie: 353
- Protein: 13g
- Fat: 10.5g
- Carbohydrates: 51g

Liquid Nutrition Smoothie

Servings: 2
Preparation time: 4 minutes

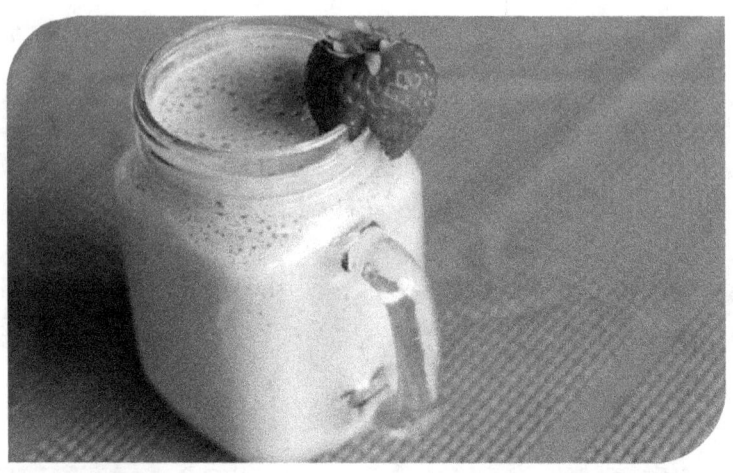

Ingredients

- 2 cups of rice milk or almond milk
- 2 to 4 tbsp of plant-based protein powder
- ½ cup blueberries or mixed berries
- 1 banana
- ½ cup chopped mango, peach or pear
- ½ cup of ice
- 1 teaspoon of coconut nectar or raw honey
- ½ to 1 cup fresh spinach

Steps to Cook

1. Mix all ingredients in a blender until the mixture is smooth and no lumps remain.
1. Pour into two glasses and enjoy.

Nutritional Information:

- Calorie: 646
- Protein: 23.3g
- Fat: 36.6g
- Carbohydrates: 64.9g

Oatmeal Pancakes With Honey and Strawberries

Servings: 1-2
Preparation time: 10 minutes
Cook time: 2-10 minutes

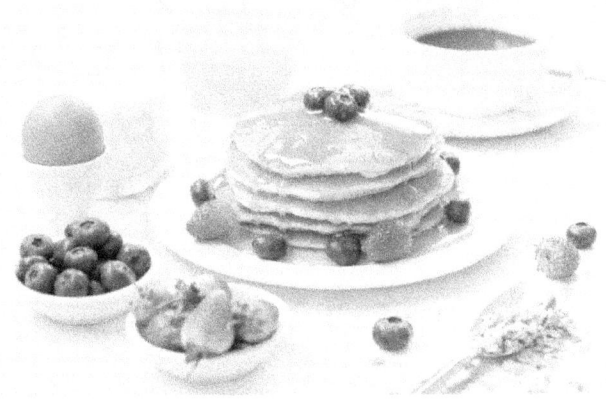

Ingredients

- 1 cup traditional oatmeal
- 1 tsp of Ground Gourmet Cinnamon
- 2 eggs
- 20 g of coconut oil
- 8 strawberries
- ¼ cup of milk
- 1 tsp of Gourmet Vanilla Essence
- Sweetener (to taste)

Steps to Cook

1. In a processor or blender put all the ingredients, except the eggs and the coconut oil. Mix for a minute or two until everything is well integrated.
2. Then add the eggs and mix again for a few seconds until it becomes a homogeneous mass.
3. Heat a large skillet, add the coconut oil and wait for it to melt. Put a medium ladle of mixture on the pancake and cook until bubbles begin to appear on the top side; turn and cook on the other side until golden brown.
4. Remove from the pan and keep covered until all the mixture is finished. Reheat in the oven if necessary.
5. Garnish with strawberries and serve accompanied by berries and maple syrup or honey as desired.

Nutritional Information:

- Calorie: 91.4
- Protein: 3.7g
- Fat: 3.7g
- Carbohydrates: 11.9g

Protein Smoothie of Pear, Apple And Banana

Servings: 2
Preparation time: 4 minutes

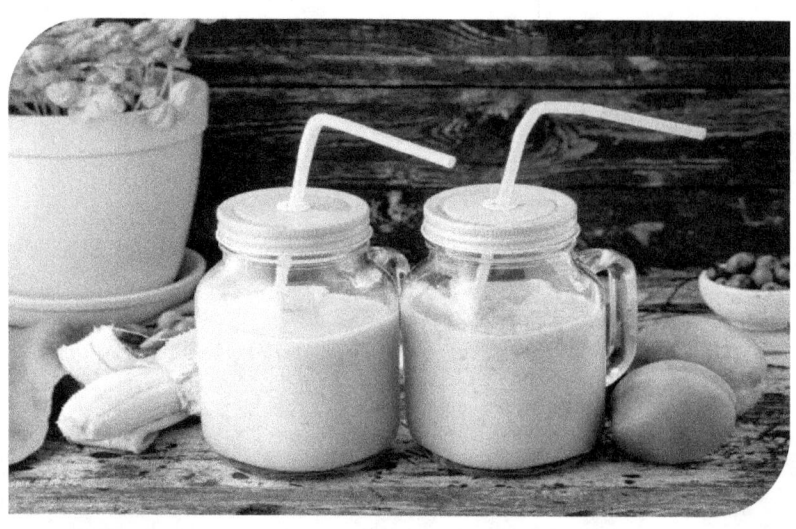

Ingredients

- 1 pear
- ½ glass water
- 1 banana
- 9 ice cubes
- 1 apple
- Sweetener to taste

Steps to Cook

1. Wash the pear well and cut it into cubes with the peel and everything, peel and cut the banana and the apple
2. Put the chopped fruit in the blender and add the water and the 9 ice cubes
3. Once it begins to liquefy, turn off the blender uncover and add the sweetener I added a jet
4. Whisk a little more until the ice and fruit are well crushed
5. Now to enjoy it! It is fresh, creamy and above all delicious

Nutritional Information:

- Calorie: 290.7
- Protein: 3.9g
- Fat: 1.3g
- Carbohydrates: 73.6g

Smoothie of Pear And Banana

Servings: 3-4
Preparation time: 4 minutes

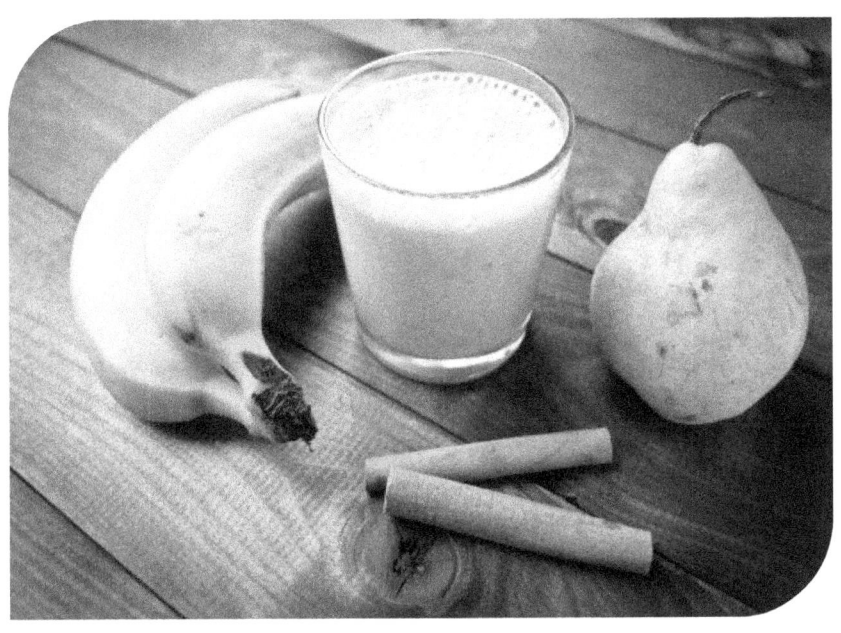

Ingredients

- 2 cups of pear juices
- 2 ripe bananas
- Sugar to taste or artificial sweetener
- 2 cups of ice cubes

Steps to Cook

1. Put the banana cut into pieces, pear juices and ice cubes in the blender glass.
2. Blend at maximum speed until everything is integrated.
3. Serve immediately in tall glasses and drink preferably immediately so that they do not lose their properties.

Nutritional Information:

- Calorie: 208.3
- Protein: 11.1g
- Fat: 6g
- Carbohydrates: 30.7g

Pineapple Kefir Smoothie

Servings: 2
Preparation time: 4 minutes

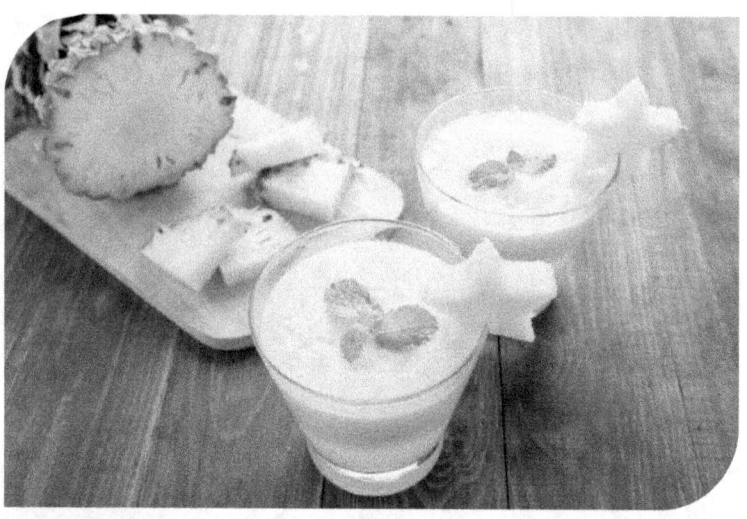

Ingredients

- 1 cup kefir
- 1 slice pineapple
- Ice to taste

Steps to Cook

1. Cut the pineapple slice into small pieces, removing the heart.
2. Put the small glass of the blender, add the kefir and blend.
3. Serve with ice to taste.

Nutritional Information:

- Calorie: 111
- Protein: 3.7g
- Fat: 2.7g
- Carbohydrates: 17.9g

Green Smoothie With Fruits and Vitamins

Servings: 2
Preparation time: 4 minutes

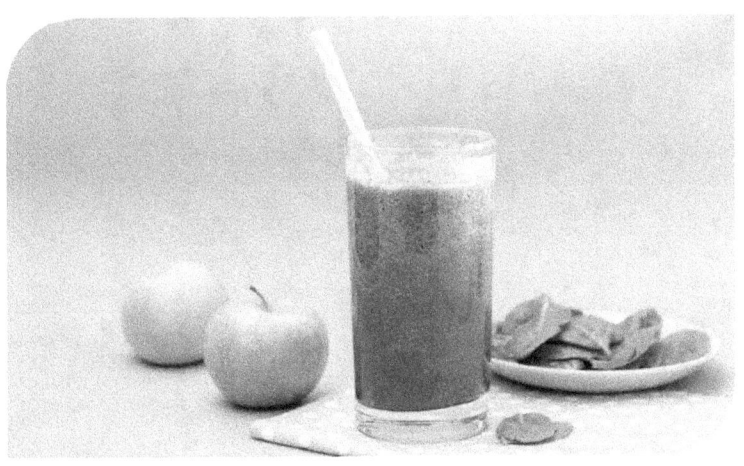

Ingredients

- ½ cucumber
- 3 tsp of maca powder
- Celery
- 1 cup of water
- 1 green apple
- 3 tsp of chia seeds

Steps to Cook

1. Pour all the ingredients in the blender and process them until you get a homogeneous drink.
2. Consume it as part of breakfast, or 30 minutes before breakfast.

Nutritional Information:

- Calorie: 184.2
- Protein: 4.3g
- Fat: 1.3g
- Carbohydrates: 44.6g

Granola, Greek Yogurt And Red Berries

Servings: 1
Preparation time: 2 minutes
Cooking: 15-20 minutes

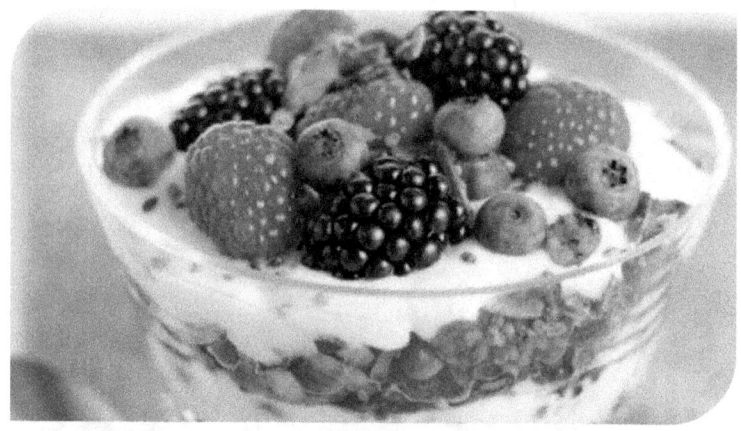

Ingredients

- 3 or 4 tbsp of granola
- 1 Greek yogurt
- 2 tbsp of red berries

Steps to Cook

For the granola:
1. Mix all ingredients in a bowl
2. Spread the mixture on a cookie sheet
3. Bake for 15-20 minutes at 180°C
4. While it is in the oven, stir it so that the whole mixture is browned equally
5. Add the granola in the glass or bowl where you are going to eat.
6. And add the yogurt and red berries.

Nutritional Information:

- Calorie: 250.9
- Protein: 14g
- Fat: 7g
- Carbohydrates: 34g

Waffles With Peanut Butter

Servings: 2
Preparation time: 2 minutes
Cooking: 15 minutes

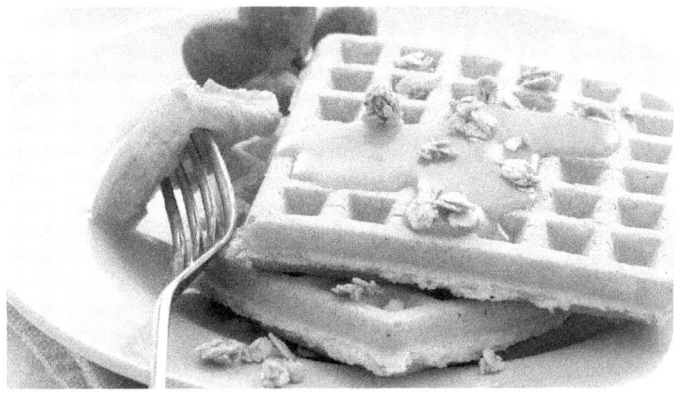

Ingredients

- ¼ lbs. of wheat flour
- 1 tbsp of baking powder
- 1 tbsp of butter
- ¼ cup of milk
- 1 tbsp of sugar
- 1 pinch of salt
- 2 tbsp peanut butter
- 1 jet of vanilla essence

Steps to Cook

1. In a bowl mix the wheat flour, the baking powder, the salt and the sugar.
2. Add the milk, vanilla essence and melted butter, mix everything very well until obtaining a homogeneous mixture.
3. Arrange the waffle dough evenly in the waffle iron, close and cook at medium temperature for 5 minutes.
4. Serve the waffles with the peanut butter, if you want to accompany it with some sliced of banana, strawberries and whipped cream, this recipe is perfect for breakfast.

Nutritional Information:

- Calorie: 333.4
- Protein: 10.3g
- Fat: 24.4g
- Carbohydrates: 16g

Chia And Mango Pudding

Servings: 2
Calories: 159
Preparation time: 10 minutes

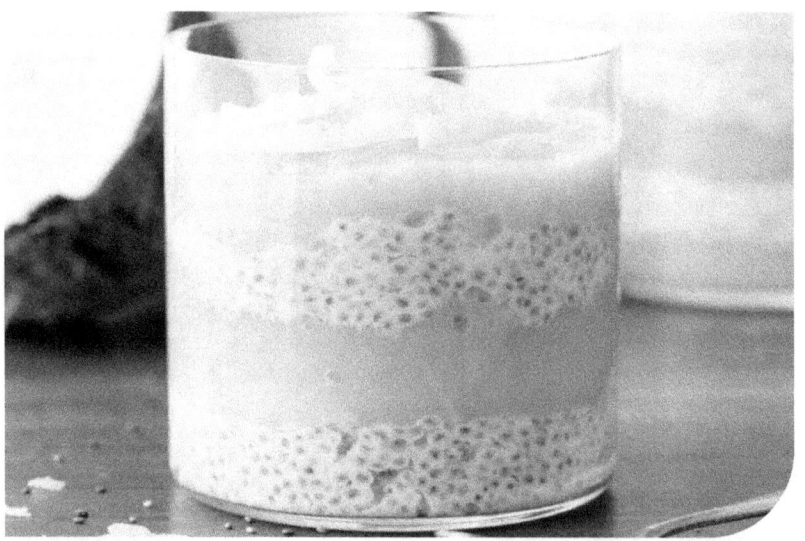

Ingredients

- 3 tsp of grated coconut
- 3 tsp of pecan nut
- 4 tbsp of chia of cinnamon
- 1 cup coconut milk
- ½ cups mango, cubed
- 1 tbsp of honey

Steps to Cook

1. Mix all the ingredients in a mason jar or on a small plate. Reserve a little coconut, walnuts and mango to decorate.
2. Refrigerate overnight or for at least 10 minutes so that the chia moistens and the preparation has a thicker consistency.
3. Decorate with grated coconut and walnut and mango pieces.

Nutritional Information:

- Calorie: 431
- Protein: 10.3g
- Fat: 27.5g
- Carbohydrates: 5.9g

Papaya Juice, Grapefruit And Nopal

Servings: 2
Calories: 156
Preparation time: 5 minutes

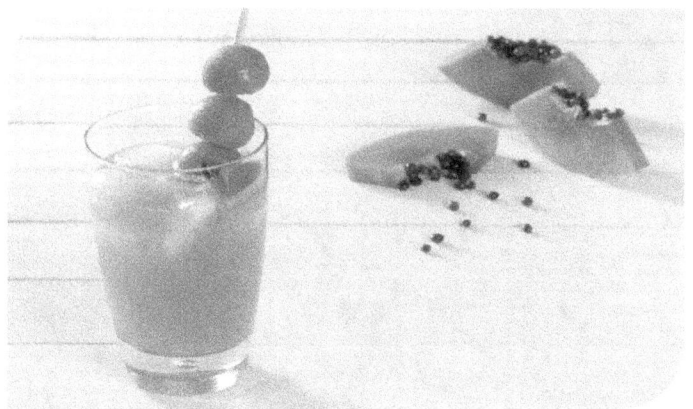

Ingredients

- ¼ nopales
- ½ cups of water
- 1 ½ oz. papaya
- 1 celery stick
- 1 ½ pineapple
- 1 grapefruit, peeled

Steps to Cook

1. Blend all the ingredients.
2. Serve.

Nutritional Information:

- Calorie: 127
- Protein: 2.1g
- Fat: 0.5g
- Carbohydrates: 32g

Avocado Sandwich And Spinach

Servings: 2
Preparation time: 5 minutes
Cooking time: 5 minutes

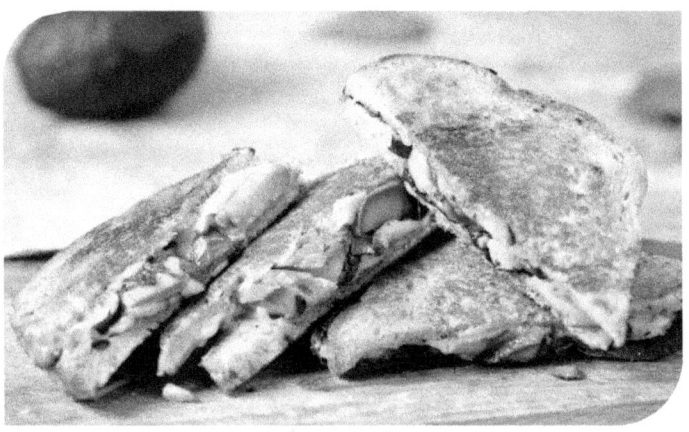

Ingredients

- 8 whole grain breads
- 4 teaspoons light mayonnaise
- 1 bunch of spinach, washed and disinfected
- 1 cup arugula, washed and disinfected
- 4 avocados, ripe
- to taste of salt and pepper

Steps to Cook

1. Preheat the oven to 360°F.
2. Place the bread on a tray and put in the oven until toasted.
3. Spread the bread with mayonnaise, place a spinach leaf, and arugula and avocado, season with salt and pepper.
4. Serve with a refreshing mint drink.

Nutritional Information:

- Calorie: 427
- Protein: 13g
- Fat: 24.8g
- Carbohydrates: 42.5g

Hummus And Avocado Cream

Servings: 6
Preparation time: 5 minutes
Cooking time: 15 minutes

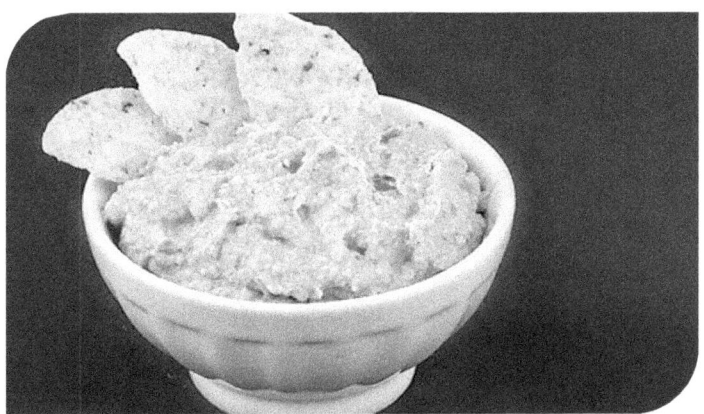

Ingredients

- ½ avocado
- 1 can of chickpeas
- 1/3 cup tahini
- ¼ cup lemon juice
- 1 garlic clove, finely chopped
- ¾ tsp whole grain salt
- ¼ tsp ground cumin
- 1 cup coriander leaves
- 2 tbsp of olive oil
- 2 tbsp coriander sprouts
- 3 bagels split in half

Steps to Cook

1. Place the avocado, chickpeas, tahini, lemon juice, garlic, salt, pepper, cumin and coriander in the processor glass.
2. Add the olive oil to the processor without stopping it in the form of a thread.
3. Process until a creamy mixture is obtained.
4. Spread some of the hummus on the bagels.
5. Top with coriander sprouts and broccoli sprouts.

Nutritional Information:

- Calorie: 60
- Protein: 2g
- Fat: 5.4g
- Carbohydrates: 4g

Portobello Tortilla

Servings: 4
Preparation time: 5 minutes
Cooking time: 10 minutes

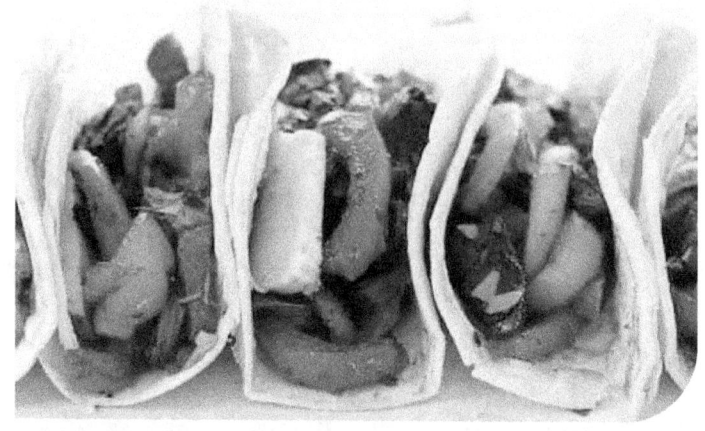

Ingredients

- ½ finely chopped onion
- 1 bell pepper
- 5 tbsp. Of olive oil
- ⅓ chopped pistachio
- ½ chopped green apple
- ½ cup hummus
- 1 tbsp. mustard
- 1 tbsp. honey bee
- 4 Portobello mushrooms
- 1 baguette
- 1 cup of quelites

Steps to Cook

1. Sauté the onion and pepper with half the oil; when they begin to brown, remove from the heat and mix with the pistachio and the apple.
2. Mix the hummus with the mustard and honey. Grill the portobello in a frying pan over medium heat with the rest of the olive oil; fill them with the pistachio mixture.
3. Toast the bread and cut it into four parts, spread a little of the prepared hummus on the base, place a portobello for each pancake and finish with the quelites.

Nutritional Information:

- Calorie: 308.8
- Protein: 14.3g
- Fat: 11.6g
- Carbohydrates: 39.5g

Chapter 2

Soups & Stews

Cabbage Soup

Servings: 2
Preparation time: 5 minutes
Cook time: 30 minutes

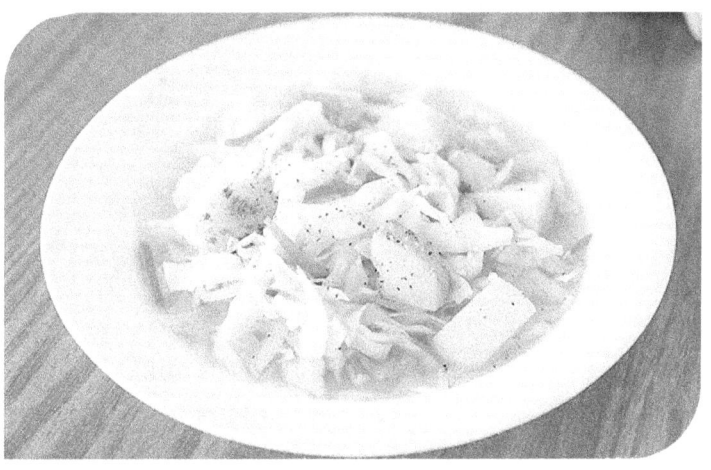

Ingredients

- 1 cabbage, chopped (small)
- 2 grated carrots
- 1 chopped onion
- 1 tablespoon of basil
- 1 tablespoon of parsley
- 1 tablespoon of oregano
- 2 celery stalks cut into slices

Steps to Cook

1. Put all the vegetables and herbs in a large soup pot, stir in tomato paste, and add water 1 to 2 inches (3 to 5 cm) below the highest level of the vegetables.
2. Cook over low heat until all the vegetables are soft (about 30 minutes).

Nutritional Information:

- Calorie: 61.9
- Protein: 2.5g
- Fat: 0.4g
- Carbohydrates: 14.1g

Sprouted Lentil And Brown Rice Stew

Servings: 2
Preparation time: 5 minutes
Cook time: 30-40 minutes

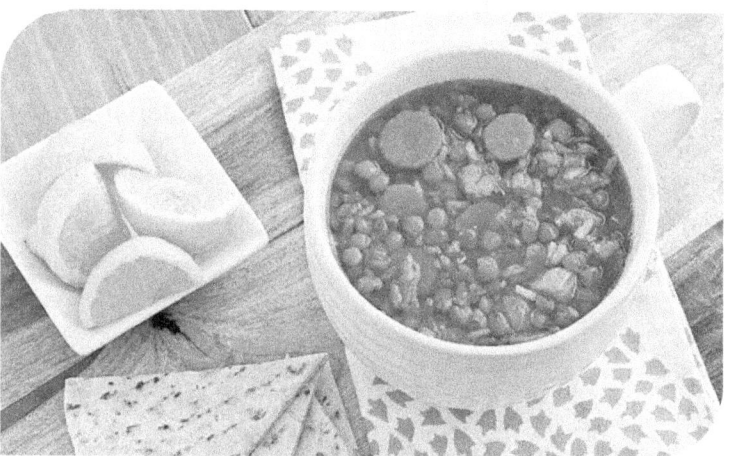

Ingredients

- 1 cup brown rice
- 1 cup black or green lentils
- 3 tablespoons of tomato puree
- 1 teaspoon salt
- 1 sweet red pepper
- 4-5 cups homemade vegetable broth
- A handful of fresh dill

Steps to Cook

1. Soak the lentils and rice together overnight in a saucepan of cool, cold water. Drain and rinse them in the morning. To keep them soaking, leave them in the strainer, at room temperature, until the germ breaks the wall.
2. Chop the sweet red pepper.
3. Once sprouted or just soaked overnight, add all ingredients except fresh dill to a saucepan. Leave them on the stove until they start to boil. Put them to cook for about 30 to 40 minutes. Stop the flame or temperature and leave them covered on the stove for another 10 minutes.
4. Chop the fresh dill and add it, stirring gently.

Nutritional Information:

- Calorie: 129.7
- Protein: 3.4g
- Fat: 5g
- Carbohydrates: 19g

Corn And Jalapeno Soup

Servings: 2
Preparation time: 5 minutes
Cook time: 4 minutes

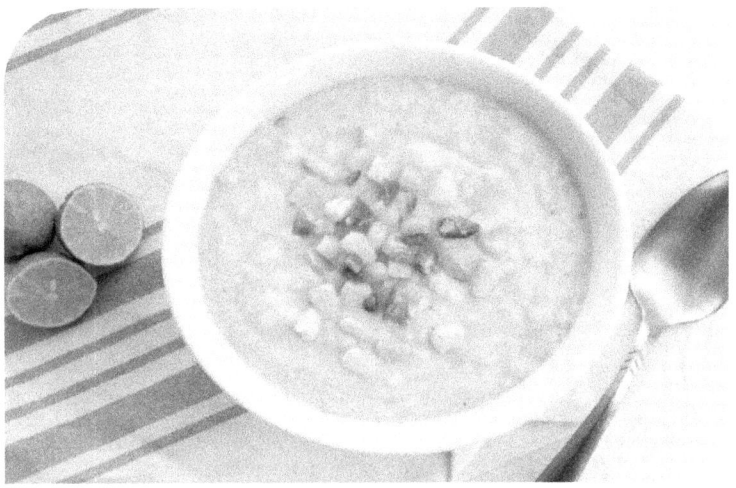

Ingredients

- ¼ cup margarine
- 2 tablespoons pickled jalapeño peppers, finely chopped
- 1 garlic clove, finely minced
- 14.75 oz. corn with cream, undrained
- 1 cup of water
- 1 tablespoon of vegetable Broth

Steps to Cook

1. Melt the margarine in a 3-liter saucepan over medium heat and fry the jalapeños and garlic, stirring frequently, for a minute.
2. Add the rest of the ingredients and cook, stirring occasionally, for 4 minutes.

Nutritional Information:

- Calorie: 125
- Protein: 5g
- Fat: 3g
- Carbohydrates: 24g

Red Pepper Cream Soup

Servings: 2-4
Preparation time: 5 minutes
Cook time: 15 minutes

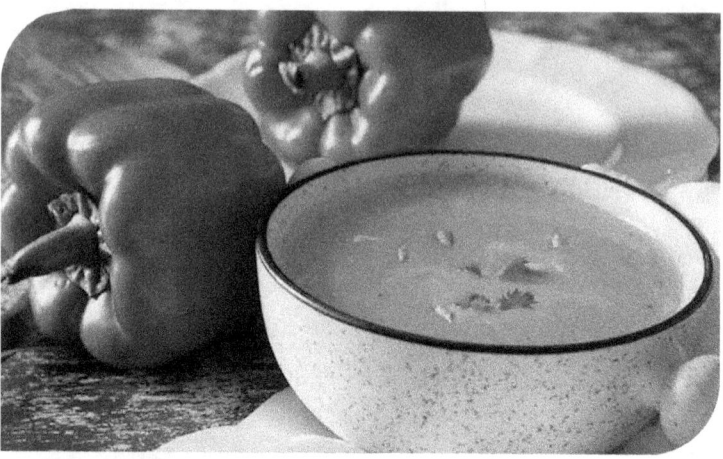

Ingredients

- 400 g red pepper without skin
- 400 g mushrooms, sliced
- 1 chopped onion
- 1 garlic clove, minced
- 2 tbsp margarine
- ½ cup soy milk
- 2 tablespoons rosemary
- 1 tbsp paprika
- 2 cups vegetable broth
- Salt, pepper, lemon juice, chopped parsley to taste
- Soy yogurt

Steps to Cook

1. Fry the onion in a large saucepan with half the margarine until glassy.
2. Add the mushrooms and garlic, along with the rosemary and sauté until the mushrooms are tender.
3. Add the pepper and the vegetable broth.
4. Cook over low heat for 15 minutes
5. Puree the previous preparation.
6. Add the lemon juice, salt and pepper to taste.
7. Serve with a little soy yogurt and chopped parsley.

Nutritional Information:

- Calorie: 220
- Protein: 4.5g
- Fat: 16g
- Carbohydrates: 16g

Pumpkin Soup

Servings: 2-4
Preparation time: 5 minutes
Cook time: 20 minutes

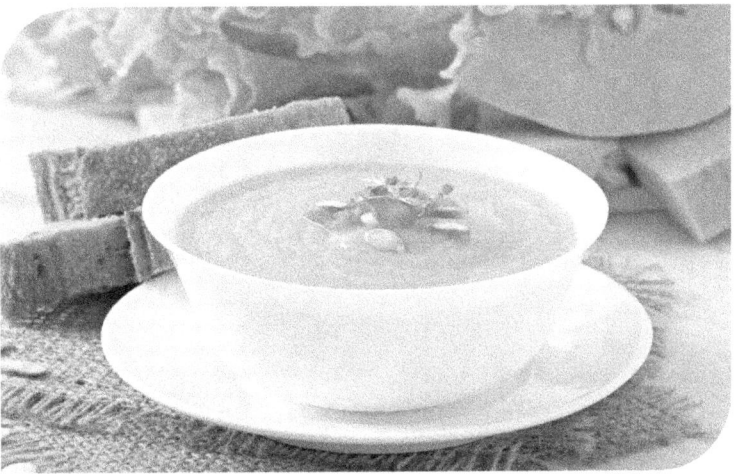

Ingredients

- ¼ lbs. of pumpkin
- ½ onion
- 1 cube of vegetable broth
- Pinch of white pepper
- Nutmeg
- Olive oil

Steps to Cook

1. Wash and peel the pumpkin and cut it into cubes.
2. Cut the onion into strips and cook for 20 minutes in water with the pumpkin, the vegetable stock, the nutmeg, the olive oil and the salt.
3. When everything is soft, run it through the mixer and add the white pepper.

Nutritional Information:

- Calorie: 34
- Protein: 1.3g
- Fat: 0.9g
- Carbohydrates: 5.1g

Corn Chowder

Servings: 2-4
Preparation time: 5 minutes
Cook time: 30 minutes

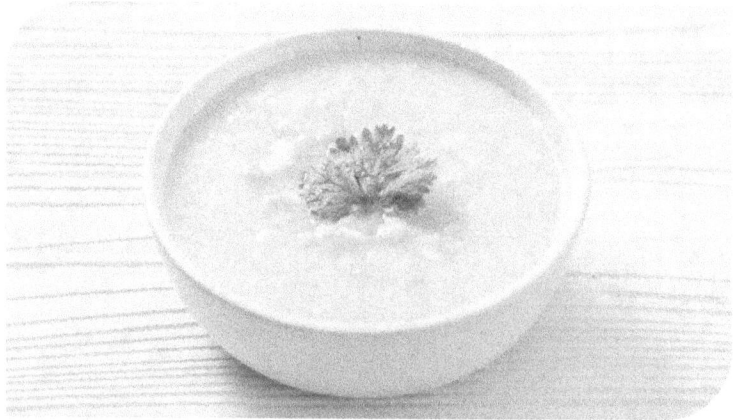

Ingredients

- 4 ears of corn
- 1 small pumpkin
- 1 grated carrot
- 1 celery branch
- 3 tbsp chopped parsley
- 2 tablespoons basil
- 1 tbsp coarse salt
- 5 tbsp of butter

Steps to Cook

1. Fill almost to the edge (leave 10 cm. So that it does not overflow) a pot with water. Add the coarse salt, the squash, washed and cut, the potatoes peeled and cut into small pieces, the grated carrot and the vegetables.
2. Cook everything 20 minutes after boiling, and add the butter and the trunks of the corn to which the grains will have been removed, leaving a little adhered to the trunk (the grains are set aside).
3. Cook 10 minutes, remove and strain. when serving incorporate the corn kernels. the vegetables left over from the cooking can be consumed as a puree. Vegetarians who eat cheese in their diets can add grated cheese. It can be decorated with peas or green beans.

Nutritional Information:

- Calorie: 34
- Protein: 1.3g
- Fat: 0.9g
- Carbohydrates: 5.1g

Nopales Soup

Servings: 2-4
Preparation time: 5 minutes
Cook time: 20 minutes

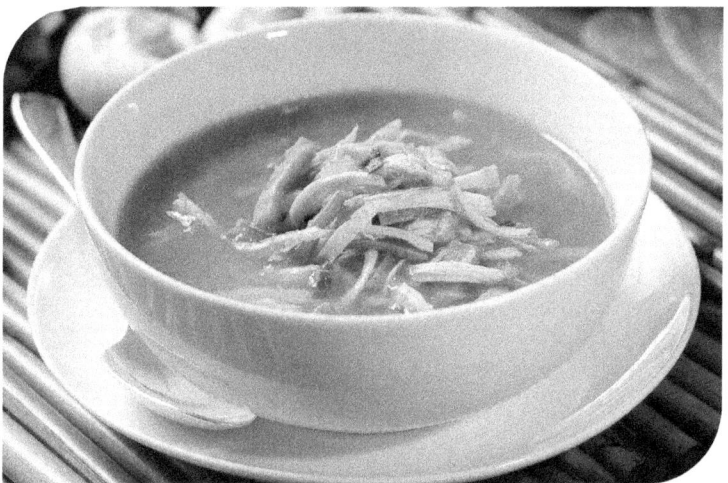

Ingredients

- 5 nopales
- 5 medium potatoes
- 6 large mushrooms
- 3 guajillo peppers
- 1 clove garlic
- 1 sprig epazote
- 1 tbsp olive oil
- Salt to taste

Steps to Cook

1. Cut the nopales into very small squares and cook them with a little salt.
2. Also divide the potatoes, in the same way, into small squares and put them to cook separately, along with the rolled mushrooms.
3. Cook the tomatoes and the chilies.
4. Prepare the sauce in the blender with the tomato and the chilies, the onion and the garlic, without straining it, fry it with a little olive oil, rinse the nopales and the potatoes, put everything in a pot and add water, salt and epazote.

Nutritional Information:

- Calorie: 107.3
- Protein: 4.2g
- Fat: 0.9g
- Carbohydrates: 24.2g

Vegetables Broth

Servings: 2-4
Preparation time: 5 minutes
Cook time: 45 minutes

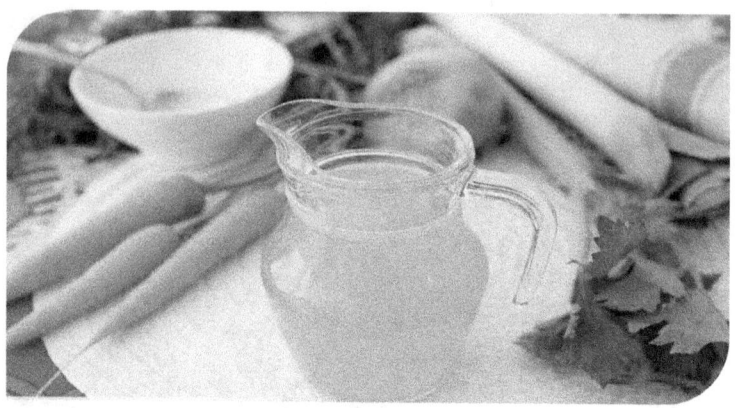

Ingredients

- 2 yellow onions, cut into slices
- 3 garlic cloves, minced
- 6 carrots, peeled and sliced
- 4 celery stalks, sliced
- 5 sprigs of dill
- 4 sprigs of parsley
- 4 chives
- 10 cups of water

Steps to Cook

1. Add the onions to a large saucepan over medium heat and stir until they release their aroma, about a minute. Add the garlic, carrots, celery, dill, parsley, and chives and cook, stirring occasionally, until the herbs release their aroma, about one minute.
2. Add the water and bring to a boil. Lower the heat, cover the pot, and simmer for about 45 minutes.
3. Add the water and bring to a boil. Lower the heat, cover the pot, and simmer for about 45 minutes.
4. Turn off the heat and let the broth cool for about 15 minutes.
5. Filter the broth through a sieve and freeze in ice cubes, or if you use it right away, pour it into glass jars. It will be kept for about a week.

Nutritional Information:

- Calorie: 107.3
- Protein: 4.2g
- Fat: 0.9g
- Carbohydrates: 24.2g

Green Soup

Servings: 2-4
Preparation time: 5 minutes
Cook time: 28-30 minutes

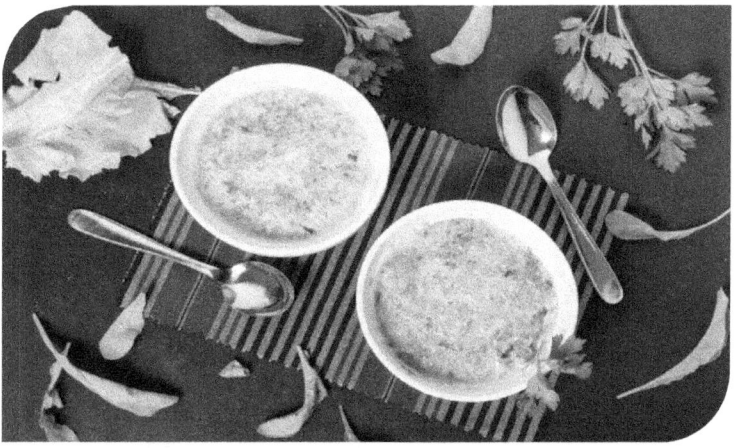

Ingredients

- 4 medium potatoes, chopped
- 5 cups of filtered water
- 1 large carrot, diced
- ½ large onion, diced thick
- ¼ bunch celery, diced thick
- 4 garlic cloves, minced
- ¼ bunch chopped kale
- 1 cup chopped cabbage
- 1-inch fresh ginger, minced
- ¼ bunch coriander

Steps to Cook

1. In a saucepan over medium heat, cook the onion and garlic in 4 tablespoons of filtered water for 2-3 minutes.
2. Add carrots, celery, and potatoes, and the rest of the filtered water.
3. Bring to a boil, keeping the stove on medium heat and stirring frequently.
4. Cook for about 10 minutes or until the vegetables have softened.
5. Add the chard, kale, coriander, and cumin, and simmer for 15 minutes.
6. Mix with an immersion blender until the soup is creamy.

Nutritional Information:

- Calorie: 90
- Protein: 4g
- Fat: 3g
- Carbohydrates: 11g

Simple Vegan Miso Soup

Servings: 3
Preparation time: 10 minutes
Cooking time: 5 minutes

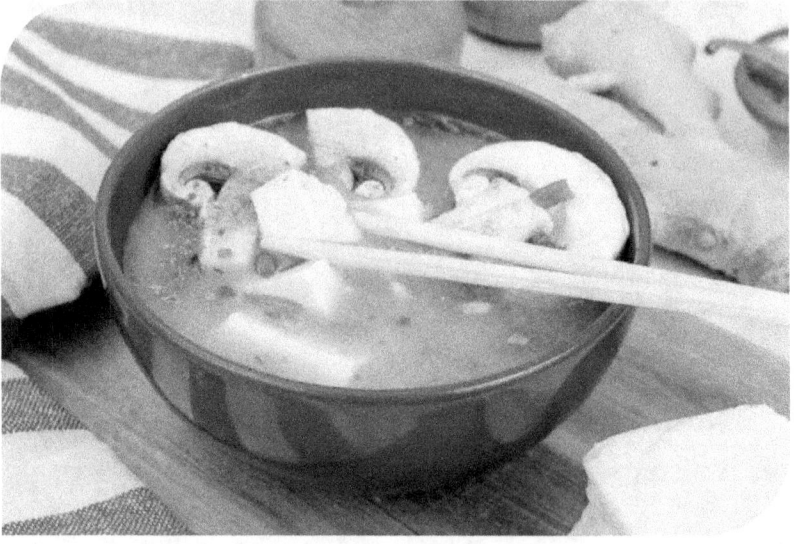

Ingredients

- ½ oz. of noodles
- 3 tablespoons of miso
- 5 cups of water
- 1 tablespoon of wakame seaweed
- 3 oz. soft tofu
- ½ cup chives

Steps to Cook

1. Cook the noodles or type of pasta you use by following the directions on the package.
2. Put the miso in a bowl. Reservation.
3. Pour the water into a pot and when it starts to boil add a little water to the bowl in which you had the miso. Stir until dissolved. Reservation.
4. Put the wakame seaweed in the pot and cook over medium high heat for about 5 minutes.
5. Remove the pot from the heat, add the water and miso mixture that you had in the bowl, the chopped tofu and the chives and stir. Remember that miso should not be heated, otherwise it loses its properties.
6. Add the cooked noodles at the end.

Nutritional Information:

- Calorie: 77.7
- Protein: 5.9g
- Fat: 2.2g
- Carbohydrates: 8.5g

Zucchini Cream With Tofu

Servings: 2-4
Preparation time: 15 minutes
Cook time: 20 minutes

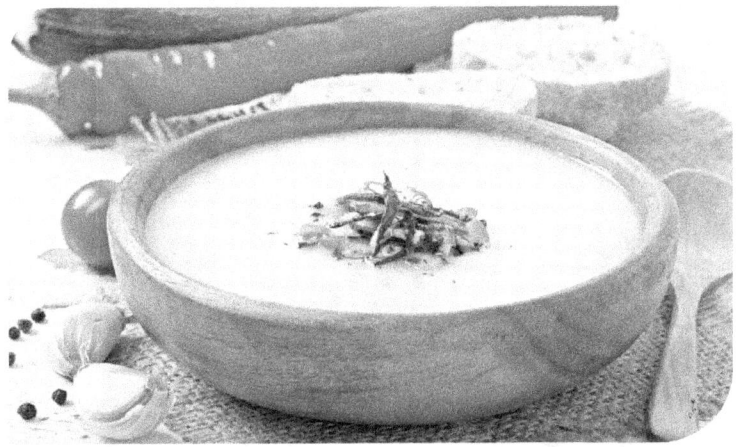

Ingredients

- 2 lbs. zucchini
- ½ lbs. tofu
- ½ lbs. carrot
- ½ lbs. leek
- Pepper
- Oil
- ¼ Garlic
- Chilli

Steps to Cook

1. Cut the leek, carrot and peeled zucchini into slices
2. Sauté the garlic, leek, chilli and carrot, when it is a little golden add the zucchini, salt and pepper to taste. Add the tofu, mixing everything well
3. Add a little water and cook until everything is soft
4. Finally go through the mixer and serve very hot

Nutritional Information:

- Calorie: 78.7
- Protein: 1.6g
- Fat: 4.7g
- Carbohydrates: 8.8g

Carrot Cream With Ginger

Servings: 4
Preparation time: 10 minutes
Cooking time: 25 minutes

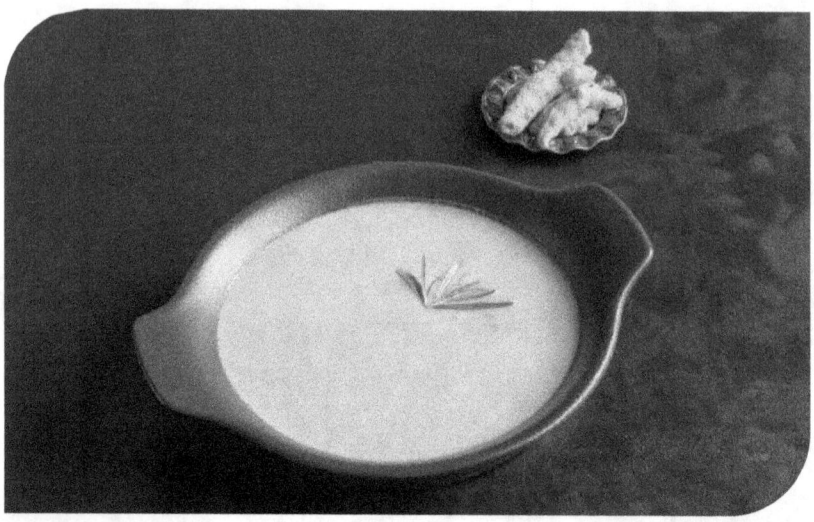

Ingredients

- 2 tbsp of canola oil
- 1 medium onion, chopped
- 1 kilo of carrots, diced
- 2 tsp grated ginger powder
- 1 liter of vegetable broth
- ½ liter of light cream
- 1 handful of pistachios
- 1 handful of coriander
- Salt and pepper to taste

Steps to Cook

1. Heat the oil in a large saucepan over medium heat.
2. Add onion and sauté until smooth and transparent, about 5 minutes.
3. Stir in the carrots, ginger, and vegetable stock, and cook over low heat for 20 minutes or until the carrots have softened.
4. Remove from the heat and let cool slightly.
5. Blend the soup until pureed and return it to the pot.
6. Add the cream and heat the soup again without letting it boil, and season with salt and pepper.
7. Separately, cut and brown the pistachios in a pan.
8. Serve the soup with the pistachios and coriander leaves.

Nutritional Information:

- Calorie: 153
- Protein: 4.3g
- Fat: 6.1g
- Carbohydrates: 22.2g

Red Lentil Hummus Cream

Servings: 2-4
Preparation time: 15 minutes
Cook time: 15-20 minutes

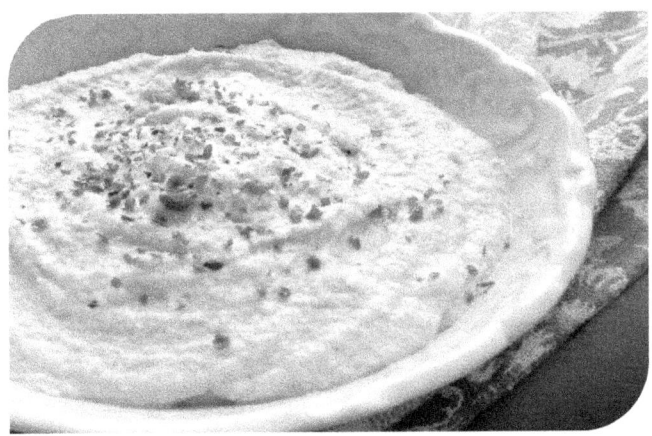

Ingredients

- ½ cup cooked red lentils
- 1 tablespoon of tahin or sesame paste
- 1 clove garlic
- 2 tablespoons of olive oil
- 2 fresh parsley sprigs
- 1 teaspoon of curry
- Salt, pepper and paprika to taste

Steps to Cook

1. For this recipe you can use a can of cooked lentils or cook them yourself at home. If you prefer the second option. Soak the lentils overnight and cook them with twice the volume of water (if you are going to make half a cup of lentils you should cook it with a cup of water)
2. Place the cooked lentils, the tahin, the garlic, the olive oil, the parsley and the spices in the glass of the blender or food processor.
3. Process until all the ingredients are well integrated and pour the preparation into a bowl.
4. You are ready to serve!

Nutritional Information:

- Calorie: 155.7
- Protein: 6.7g
- Fat: 8.6g
- Carbohydrates: 14.2g

Homemade Vegan Mayonnaise

Servings: 2-4
Preparation time: 5 minutes
Cook time: 5 minutes

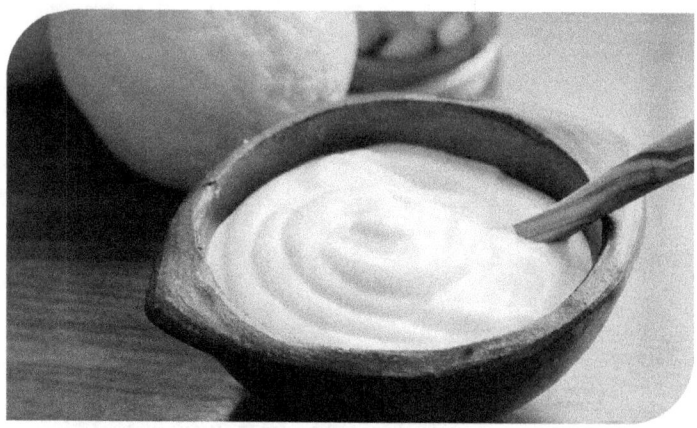

Ingredients

- 1 cup olive oil
- 1 tbsp of mustard
- ¼ cup chickpea cooking water
- 1 tsp salt
- 1 tbsp of apple cider vinegar
- **Optional**: lemon juice/juice

Steps to Cook

1. Place the chickpea water in a saucepan and bring to medium heat until it boils.
2. Boil for a few minutes until the liquid reduces a little and its consistency becomes slimy.
3. Remove from the heat, place the liquid in a bowl and let cool. Once it is cold, pour it into the glass of the blender or kitchen robot together with the mustard, salt and vinegar.
4. Blend well until all the ingredients are integrated.
5. Finally add the oil little by little while the blender continues to run.
6. Adjust the amount of salt and mustard.
7. Store in a tightly closed glass container in the refrigerator.

Nutritional Information:

- Calorie: 62.4
- Protein: 0.1g
- Fat: 7g
- Carbohydrates: 0.3g

Cauliflower Cream And Coconut Milk

Servings: 2-4
Preparation time: 5 minutes
Cook time: 5 minutes

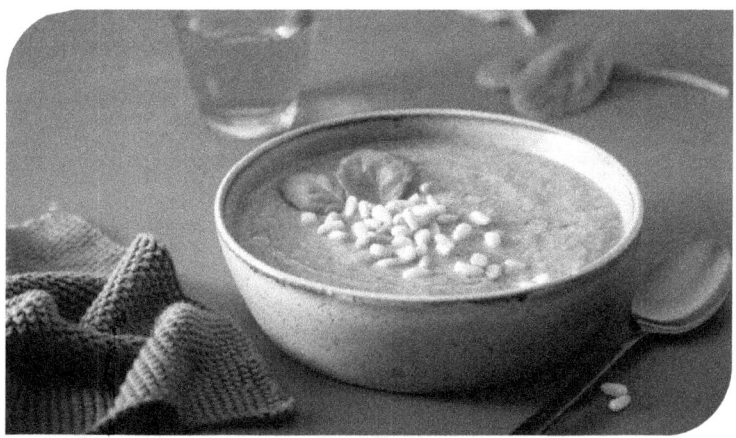

Ingredients

- 1 small cooked eggplant
- 1 cup cooked cauliflower
- 1 cup coconut milk or cream
- 1 teaspoon green curry
- Salt and pepper to taste
- Brewer's yeast and seeds for garnish

Steps to Cook

1. Place the cooked and diced eggplant, cauliflower, coconut milk, curry, salt and pepper in a blender.
2. Process well until a homogeneous cream consistency is achieved
3. Serve in a bowl and garnish with brewer's yeast, poppy and sunflower seeds.

Nutritional Information:

- Calorie: 119.9
- Protein: 2.9g
- Fat: 9.5g
- Carbohydrates: 6.9g

Split Pea Soup Recipe

Servings: 2
Preparation time: 5 minutes
Cooking time: 15-20 minutes

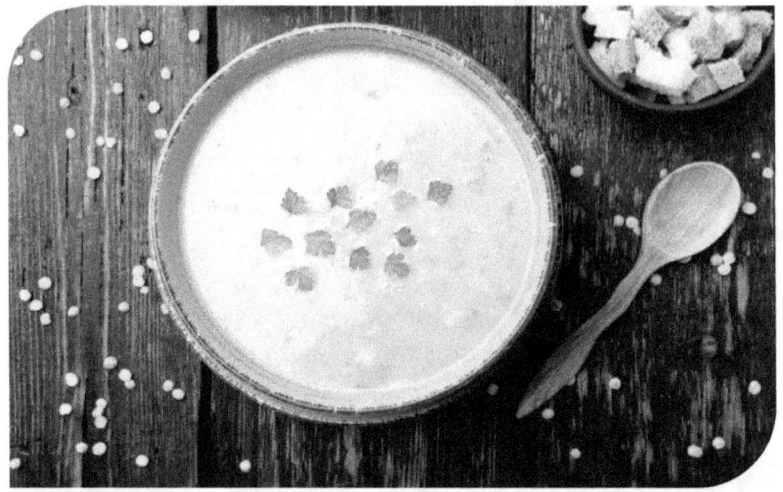

Ingredients

- 2 ½ cups green split peas
- 4 potatoes
- 1 carrot
- 2 stalks celery
- 1 coriander bouquet
- 2 wide coriander leaves
- 1 large red onion, cut into eighths
- 4 malagueta grains
- 1 ½ teaspoons of salt
- 7 cups of boiling water
- 4 tbsp of olive oil
- ½ teaspoon of pepper

Steps to Cook

1. Place the peas, potatoes, carrots, celery, coriander, cilantro, onion, malagueta and a teaspoon of salt in a pressure cooker or slow cooker.
2. Add boiling water.
3. Cook over medium heat until vegetables soften (15-20 min). Stir regularly so that it does not stick, it is better to be a cast iron or aluminum pot.

Nutritional Information:

- Calorie: 190
- Protein: 12.8g
- Fat: 0.8g
- Carbohydrates: 34.3g

Noodle soup with broccoli and ginger

Servings: 2-4
Preparation time: 5 minutes
Cook time: 10-12 minutes

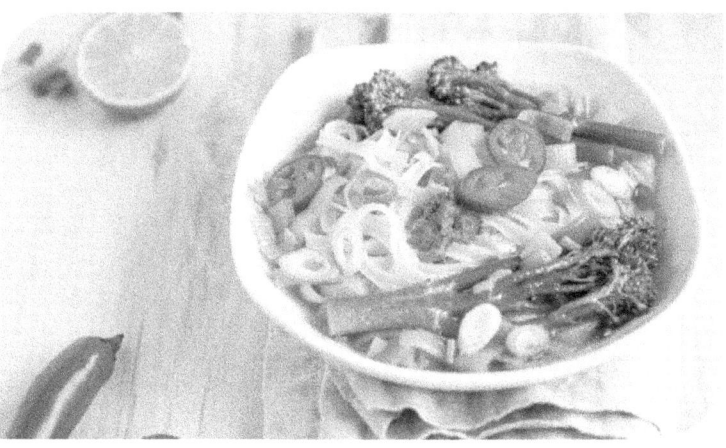

Ingredients

- 7 cups broccoli
- 12 ounces noodles
- 16 ounces firm tofu
- 2 two-inch (5 cm) pieces of seaweed wakame or alaria
- ¾ cup of wheat-free or regular tamari
- 2 medium onions, diced
- 4 tablespoons fresh ginger root, minced or finely grated
- 3 tablespoons of mirin
- 6 medium carrots
- 2 cups medium parsnips, diced

Steps to Cook

1. Separate the stems of the broccoli from their heads. Remove the outer hard layer from the stems and cut them into small bite-size pieces. Set them aside.
2. Separate the heads of the broccoli into small pieces and set them aside.
3. Cook the noodles, strain them and let them cool down. Set them aside.
4. Sauté the tofu in a nonstick skillet for 3 to 4 minutes. Add 4 teaspoons of tamari and sauté for another 3 to 4 minutes. Set it aside.
5. Place the wakame or alaria seaweed in 4 liters of water and bring them to a boil.
6. Lower the heat to medium, add the onions and cook for 10 minutes.
7. Remove the vegetables from the sea, cut them into small pieces and return them to the pot.
8. Add the ginger, remaining tamari, and mirin.
9. Continue cooking over medium heat for 5 minutes.
10. Add carrots, parsnips, and broccoli stalks. Cook for 2 minutes.
11. Gently stir the noodles and stir fry tofu. Cook for 1 minute.

12. Add the broccoli heads. Simmer over low heat until broccoli is tender, about 2-3 minutes.

Nutritional Information:

- Calorie: 216
- Protein: 12.7g
- Fat: 5.7g
- Carbohydrates: 29.6g

White Garlic Soup

Servings: 2-4
Preparation time: 5 minutes
Cook time: 10-12 minutes

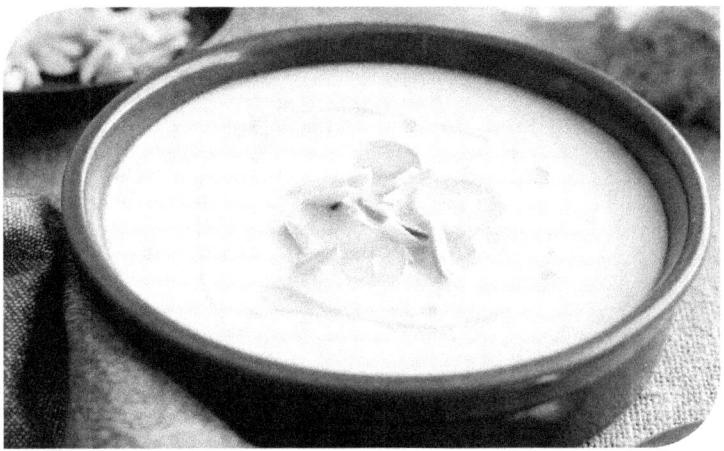

Ingredients

- 3 oz. almonds
- 2 garlic grains
- ¼ lbs. of hard white bread
- 3 oz. of extra virgin olive oil
- 5 cups of water
- 3 tablespoons sherry vinegar
- 1 bunch of muscat grapes
- Salt to taste

Steps to Cook

1. Put the bread to soak, in the liter of water, in the fridge for an hour so that it is very fresh.
2. Then the almonds are blanched with boiling water, to be able to peel them.
3. Mince the peeled garlic, peeled almonds, a little salt in a blender.
4. Then add the soaked bread and mix everything well.
5. A fine paste is made, to which add the oil slowly, so that it bonds.
6. Then add the vinegar and mix it well.
7. The fresh water is poured slowly, to mix it perfectly.
8. Place in a large bowl or in the tureen that you are going to take to the table.
9. Add the grape on top.

Nutritional Information:

- Calorie: 138.4
- Protein: 3g
- Fat: 8.8g
- Carbohydrates: 11.9g

Butternut Squash And Black Bean Chili

Servings: 2
Preparation time: 5 minutes
Cooking time: 35-40 minutes

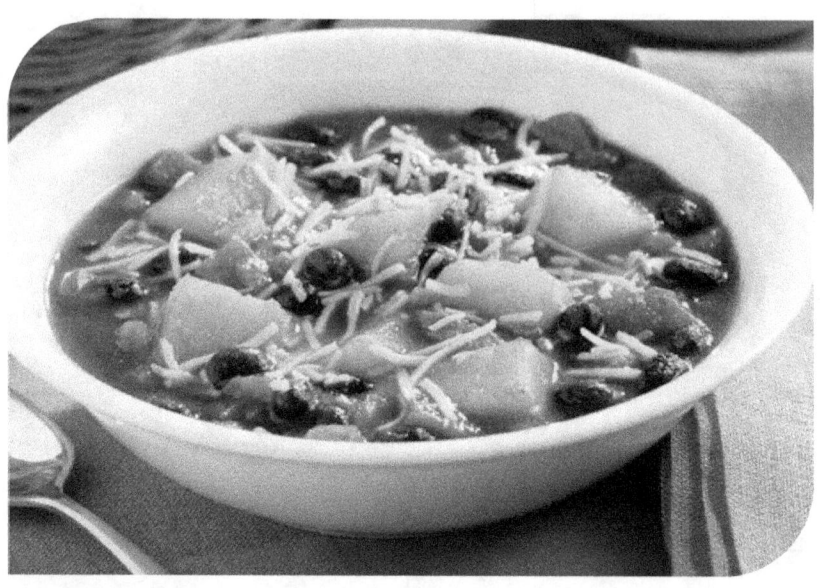

Ingredients

- ¼ cup vinaigrette
- 2 cups butternut squash
- 1 yellow onion
- 4 large garlic cloves
- 2 teaspoons of chili powder
- 1 tsp of cumin powder
- 28 oz diced tomatoes
- 15 oz black beans
- 4 green onions
- ¼ cup coriander
- ½ cup cheese

Steps to Cook

1. Heat dressing over medium heat in heavy saucepan or large deep skillet. Add the pumpkin, yellow onion and garlic; cook, stirring, for 7 minutes or until the squash is slightly soft.
2. Add the seasonings and stir for 30 seconds. Add the tomatoes and beans; bring them to a boil. Cover the pot; keep simmering over medium-low heat for 35 minutes or until squash is soft, stirring occasionally.
3. Add the green onions and coriander. Put the cheese on it.

Nutritional Information:

- Calorie: 231
- Protein: 10g
- Fat: 5g
- Carbohydrates: 38g

Sweet Potato And Carrot Soup

Servings: 2-4
Preparation time: 5 minutes
Cook time: 13 minutes

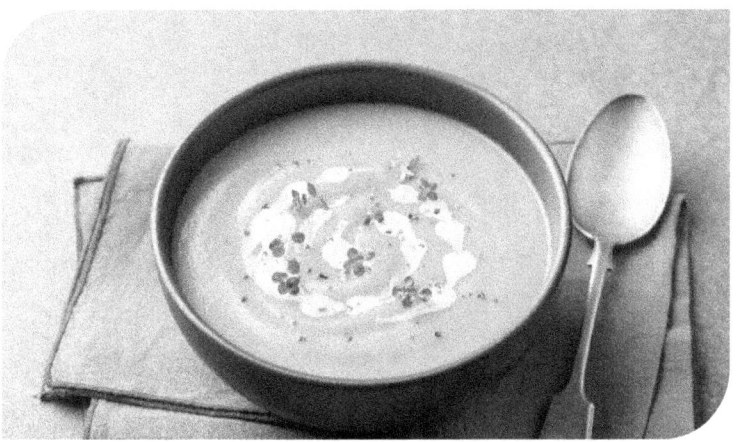

Ingredients

- 1 large onion, chopped
- 2 garlic cloves, minced
- 2 cm ginger, peeled and minced
- 2 heaping tablespoons of powdered vegetable broth
- ½ teaspoon turmeric
- 1½ pound carrots cut into small pieces
- 1 medium sweet potato, diced
- Water
- A handful of cashews

Steps to Cook

1. Heat 2 tablespoons of water in a heavy-bottom soup pot. Once it starts to sparkle, add the chopped onions. Sauté them until they become translucent, adding a tablespoon of water at a time to prevent sticking. Add the garlic and ginger and sauté for another minute.
2. Add the sweet potato, carrots, vegetable stock, and a little more boiling water than necessary to cover the vegetables. Stir well with a spoon. Bring to a boil and simmer until the vegetables are soft enough to puree, about 10 to 13 minutes.
3. Let the soup cool slightly, then add the cashews (you can soak them first) and puree them with an immersion blender or regular blender. Add a little boiled water if the soup is too thick.
4. Garnish with parsley and enjoy!

Nutritional Information:

- Calorie: 132.9
- Protein: 5.8g
- Fat: 0.7g
- Carbohydrates: 27g

Cooked Peas And Seitan

Servings: 2-4
Preparation time: 5 minutes
Cook time: 1h

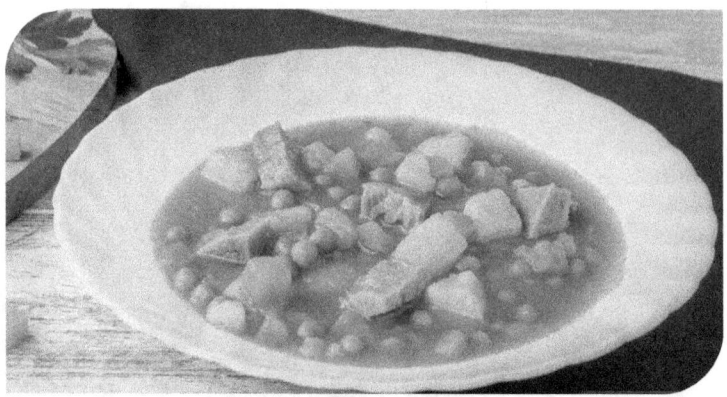

Ingredients

- ½ lbs. peas
- 3 oz. from seitan
- 1 onion.
- 1 carrot
- 2 potatoes
- Sweet paprika powder
  Oil, water and salt

Steps to Cook

1. Start by peeling and cutting the onion and frying it in the pot,
2. Then peel and cut the potatoes, the carrot and put them in the same pot together with the peas. Add water to cover all the ingredients and put it on medium heat. Also put a jet of olive oil, a pinch of salt and half a teaspoon of sweet paprika.
3. Cut the seitan into cubes and brown it a little in a frying pan and then add it to the pot with the peas. In the case that you use textured soy, it is not necessary to soak it; you can put it at the same time with the peas and the rest of the ingredients.
4. With all the ingredients in the pot, let them cook over medium heat. It will take an hour or so for the broth to reduce and get a little fat.

Nutritional Information:

- Calorie: 132.9
- Protein: 5.8g
- Fat: 0.7g
- Carbohydrates: 27g

Bimi Cream

Servings: 2-4
Preparation time: 5 minutes
Cook time: 8-10 minutes

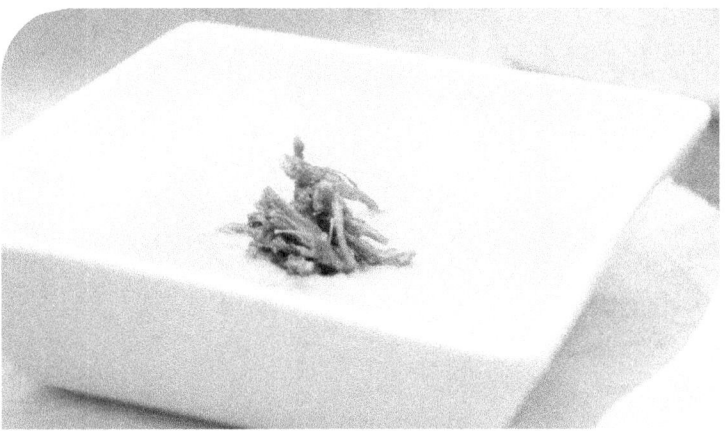

Ingredients

- ¼ lbs. Bimi
- ¼ lbs. potato
- 1 red onion
- 2 cloves of garlic
- Salt
- Pepper
- Extra virgin olive oil

Steps to Cook

1. Peel and cut the onion and the garlic cloves. Put a splash of oil in the pot and when it is hot add the garlic until it is slightly brown. Also put the chopped onion with a little salt and pepper. Let simmer until softened. Add the bimi and cut and let it make about 2 or 3 minutes.
2. Then add the diced potatoes and cover with water. If you make it in a traditional pot, leave until the potato is ready.
3. Now all that remains is to beat all the ingredients until you have a smooth and homogeneous cream.
4. One presentation idea for bimi cream is to reserve several bimi stems and grill them 3-4 minutes just before serving.

Nutritional Information:

- Calorie: 54
- Protein: 6g
- Fat: 1g
- Carbohydrates: 1g

Broccoli And Almonds Cream

Servings: 2-4
Preparation time: 5 minutes
Cook time: 5 minutes

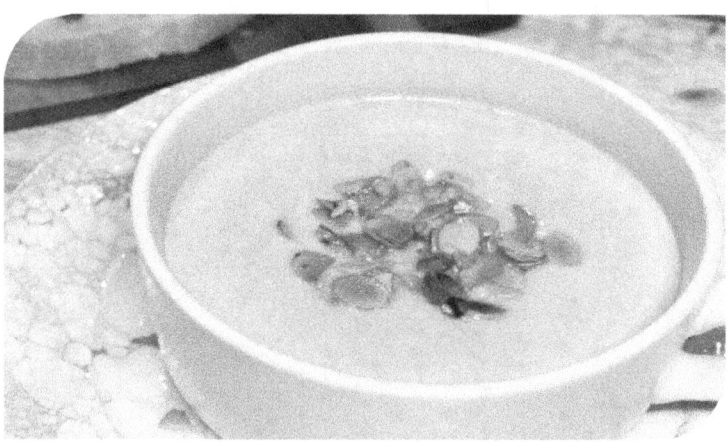

Ingredients

- 2 broccolis
- 3 tablespoons of almond powder
- 2 cloves of garlic
- 1 onion
- ½ zucchini
- ¼ cup white wine
- 1 slice of bread
- Salt, pepper and oil

Steps to Cook

1. Fry the garlic, onion and zucchini in the pot, after having peeled and finely chopped them for about three or four minutes. Then add the wine and leave it on the fire for another minute.
2. While you are cutting and cleaning the stems of the broccoli and then add it to the pot with the onion, zucchini and garlic. Add enough water to cover all the ingredients and once it begins to boil, let it cook for about 5 minutes.
3. Remove from the heat and add the slightly crumbled bread, the tablespoons of almond and a pinch of salt and pepper.
4. Beat everything until fine cream remains and serve with a little olive oil.

Nutritional Information:

- Calorie: 86
- Protein: 3.6g
- Fat: 5.2g
- Carbohydrates: 5.4g

Pumpkin Cream

Servings: 2-4
Preparation time: 5 minutes
Cook time: 25-30 minutes

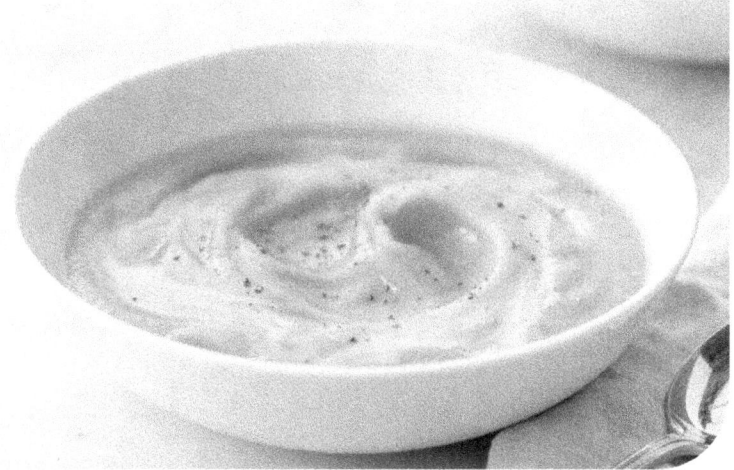

Ingredients

- *1 pumpkin*
- *2 carrots*
- *1 large potato*
- *Olive oil*
- *Nutmeg*
- *Pumpkin seeds*
- *Salt*

Steps to Cook

1. Wash and peel all the vegetables, cut them into cubes and cook them for approximately 25-30 minutes.
2. Let it warm a little and crush it well, leaving a fine texture.
3. Once you have the consistency that you like the most, add salt to taste and a splash of olive oil (if possible, be extra virgin). Add a pinch of nutmeg to give it a touch of flavor (but be careful because if you spend a bit it can give a too strong flavor).
4. When presenting, you can add some pumpkin seeds.

Nutritional Information:

- Calorie: 34
- Protein: 1.3g
- Fat: 0.9g
- Carbohydrates: 5.1g

Chestnut Cream And Boniato

Servings: 2-4
Preparation time: 5 minutes
Cook time: 50 minutes

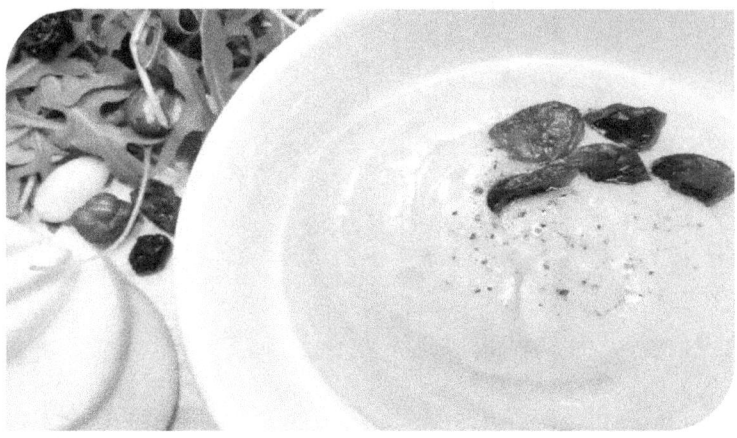

Ingredients

- ½ lbs. chestnuts
- ½ lbs. sweet potato
- 2 cups vegetable broth
- 3 oz. mushrooms
- Extra virgin olive oil
- Salt
- Pepper
- Garlic powder

Steps to Cook

1. Peel the chestnuts. Remove the thickest part of the skin, the inner part of the skin that is thinner will remain, but remove it after cooking. Put them to cook for about 30-40 minutes. Peel the sweet potato. Cut into large cubes and cook for 20-30 minutes in water.
2. Drain the chestnuts and remove the remaining skin. Drain the cooked sweet potato and put in the mixer together with the vegetable broth.
3. Once the cream is homogeneous, add a little salt and pepper and a splash of olive oil.
4. To flavor the cream sautéed mushrooms. Cut them into small cubes and put in the pan with 1 tbsp of olive oil and season with a little salt and garlic powder. Leave until golden brown.
5. Put the base with the cream and a handful of mushrooms and a little parsley.

Nutritional Information:

- Calorie: 40
- Protein: 0g
- Fat: 0g
- Carbohydrates: 9g

Carrot Mayonnaise

Servings: 4-6
Preparation time: 5 minutes

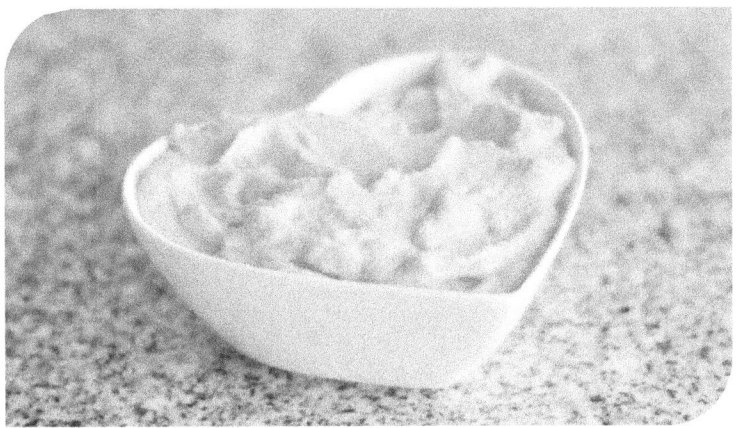

Ingredients

- 1 lb. steamed carrots
- 1 clove garlic
- Cooking liquid for carrots
- ½ lemon just the juice
- 2 tablespoons oil
- 1 pinch sea salt

Steps to Cook

1. Blend the carrots and garlic, adding the necessary cooking liquid until obtaining a cream.
2. Remove and add the juice, oil and salt. And use.

Nutritional Information:

- Calorie: 132.9
- Protein: 5.8g
- Fat: 0.7g
- Carbohydrates: 27g

Avocado, Green Apple, Lime And Mint Cream

Servings: 2-4
Preparation time: 5 minutes

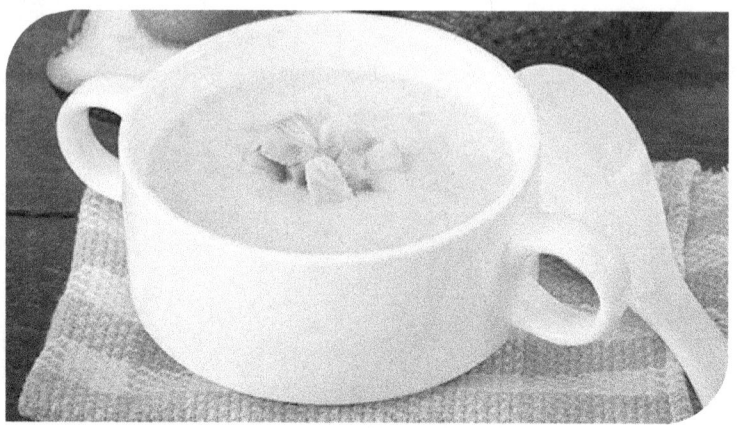

Ingredients

- 2 ripe avocados
- 1 green apple
- 1 lime
- Fresh mint
- 1 tablespoon of fine unrefined salt dessert
- 1 pinch of ground pepper
- Sesame seeds (optional)

Steps to Cook

1. Peel and remove the stone from the avocados. Chop them into not very large pieces and reserve.
2. Squeeze the lime juice. Put the avocados in the mixer glass and add the juice.
3. Cut the apple (if it is not organic, better peel it). Remove the seeds and the heart. Add it to the mixer.
4. Add the salt and pepper.
5. Grind until the dough is homogeneous. Wash and cut the mint leaves very thin. Add to the mixture and beat again.
6. To decorate, put some mint leaves and add the sesame seeds topping.

Nutritional Information:

- Calorie: 306
- Protein: 10g
- Fat: 15g
- Carbohydrates: 38g

Mushroom Cream

Servings: 2-4
Preparation time: 5 minutes
Cook time: 20-30 minutes

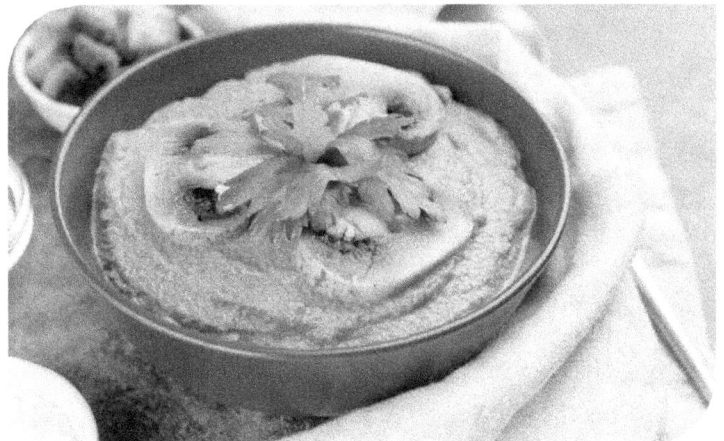

Ingredients

- ¼ lbs. of mushrooms
- ½ cauliflower (not very large)
- 1 potato
- ½ onion
- 2 tablespoons of vegetable cream
- Oil
- Salt and parsley

Steps to Cook

1. Put to cook the cauliflower and the potato, which you will remove when both are beginning to be soft. While it is done, finely chop the onion and fry it together with the mushrooms, in my case rolled. Let it simmer until all the water released by the mushrooms is consumed and the onion is soft.
2. It only remains to beat everything. Start with the cream with the potato and the cauliflower, which previously drained a little, but without throwing the broth, in case later you need to correct the thickness of the cream. Then gradually add the mushrooms and continued beating until a fine cream remained.
3. Reserve some fried mushrooms for the presentation, with a few drops of olive oil and a little parsley.

Nutritional Information:

- Calorie: 241
- Protein: 4.1g
- Fat: 16g
- Carbohydrates: 21g

Lombarda Cream

Servings: 2-4
Preparation time: 5 minutes
Cook time: 25 minutes

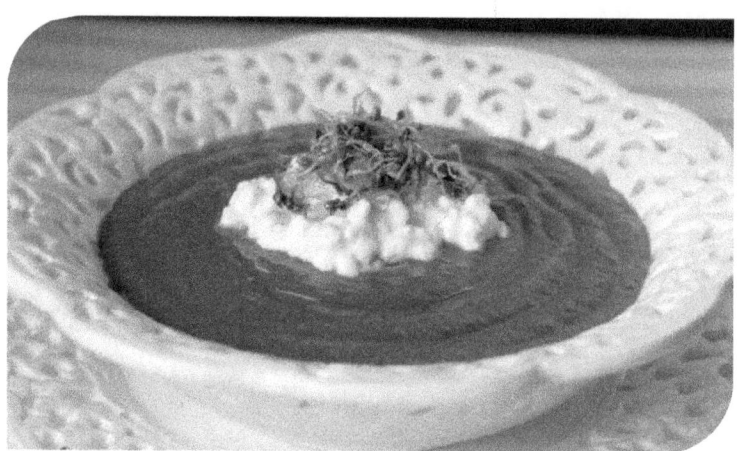

Ingredients

- ½ red cabbage
- 1 leek
- ½ onion
- 2 small potatoes
- Vegetable soy cream
- Salt
- Kale chips
- Fried onion

Steps to Cook

1. First of all, wash and cut the vegetables into not very large pieces. Put the leek to sauté in olive oil and add the red cabbage. Add a little salt and let it cook for about 10 minutes. Then add the potatoes and cover everything with water.
2. Let it boil for about 15 minutes and then remove from the heat.
3. Pass it through a mixer and add a splash of vegetable cream and correct salt to taste. At the time of serving add the kale chips and the fried onion.

Nutritional Information:

- Calorie: 27
- Protein: 1g
- Fat: 0g
- Carbohydrates: 3g

Potato Soup

Servings: 2-4
Preparation time: 5 minutes
Cook time: 20-25 minutes

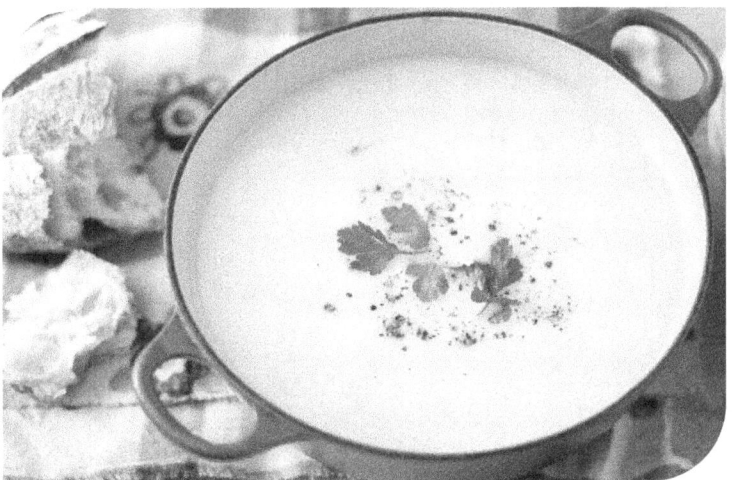

Ingredients

- 6 medium yellow potatoes
- ½ cup white miso
- 1 ½ tbsp garlic powder
- ⅓ cup nutritional yeast
- 1 ½ tablespoon Herbs de Provence seasoning
- ½ cup soy milk

Steps to Cook

1. Wash, clean and chop the potatoes into large pieces and put them in a medium saucepan.
2. Add enough water to cover the potatoes and bring to a boil. Cook the potatoes over low heat until soft.
3. Turn off the heat and, without draining, use the press to tear apart the large pieces of potato. For a softer, creamier soup, mash the potato longer or use an immersion chopper.
4. Add the miso, garlic powder, nutritional yeast, and Herbs de Provence seasoning; then stir or mash everything to mix completely.
5. Add a little soy milk to dilute the soup if you think it is too thick, or just to add a little more creaminess.
6. Serve it hot.

Nutritional Information:

- Calorie: 178.9
- Protein: 4g
- Fat: 6g
- Carbohydrates: 27g

Mushroom Cream Soup And Rice

Servings: 2
Preparation time: 5 minutes
Cooking time: 5-10 minutes

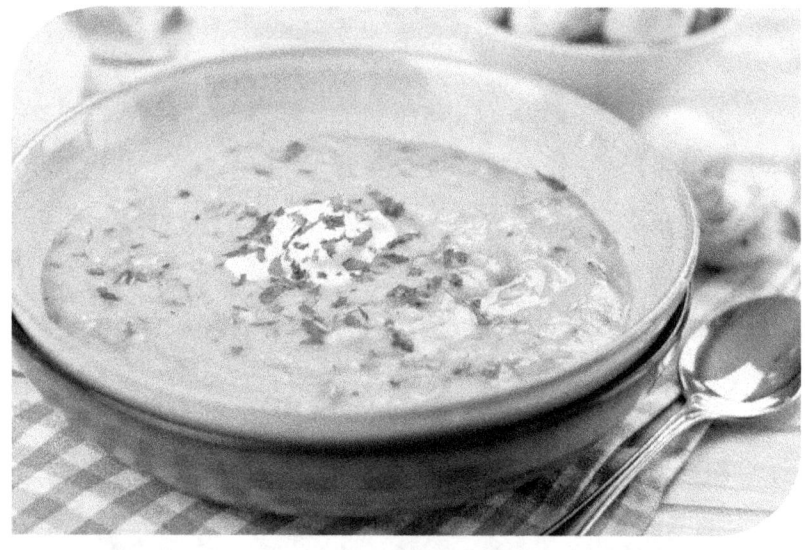

Ingredients

- ¼ lbs. of Cream Cheese
- 2 tbsp. Of olive oil
- 2 tbsp. chopped onion
- 1 garlic clove, crushed
- 1 sprig of fresh rosemary
- 2 ½ cups. filleted mushrooms
- 1 tbsp. beef broth powder
- 3 cups. of water
- Salt and pepper
- 1 cup cooked wild rice

Steps to Cook

1. Heat the olive oil in a saucepan and add garlic, onion and rosemary. Sauté a few minutes and add the mushrooms, cook.
2. Incorporate powdered broth and water. Remove the sprig of fresh rosemary.
3. Blend the above with the Cream Cheese and return to the saucepan. Wait for it to boil and rectify the seasoning with salt and pepper.

Nutritional Information:

- Calorie: 188.7
- Protein: 4g
- Fat: 7.7g
- Carbohydrates: 26.2g

Vegetable Soup

Servings: 2
Preparation time: 5 minutes
Cooking time: 25 minutes

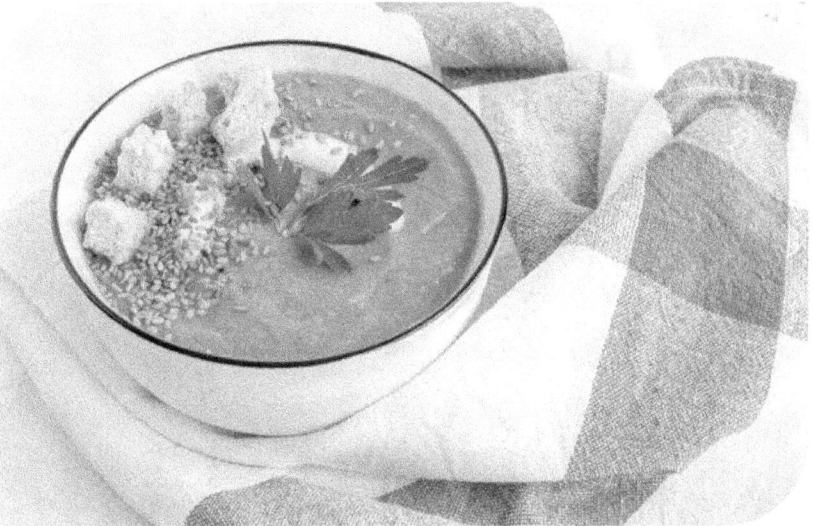

Ingredients

- 2 carrots
- 2 onions
- 2 celery stalks
- 1 head of broccoli chopped
- 2 tomatoes
- 8 mushrooms cut in half
- 3 stems of fresh parsley
- A bay leaf
- Pepper
- Salt to taste

Steps to Cook

1. The first thing you should know is that the list of ingredients is referential. You can freely include other vegetables.
2. Fill a large pot with water and bring to a boil. Add the previously cut vegetables as indicated in the recipe and simmer for about 20 to 30 minutes.
3. During this period the vegetable broth will consume the nutrients from the vegetables to create a delicious blend of flavors. Don't forget to add salt to taste before serving.

Nutritional Information:

- Calorie: 156
- Protein: 5.3g
- Fat: 2.2g
- Carbohydrates: 29.1g

Zucchinis Soup

Servings: 2
Preparation time: 5 minutes
Cooking time: 25-30 minutes

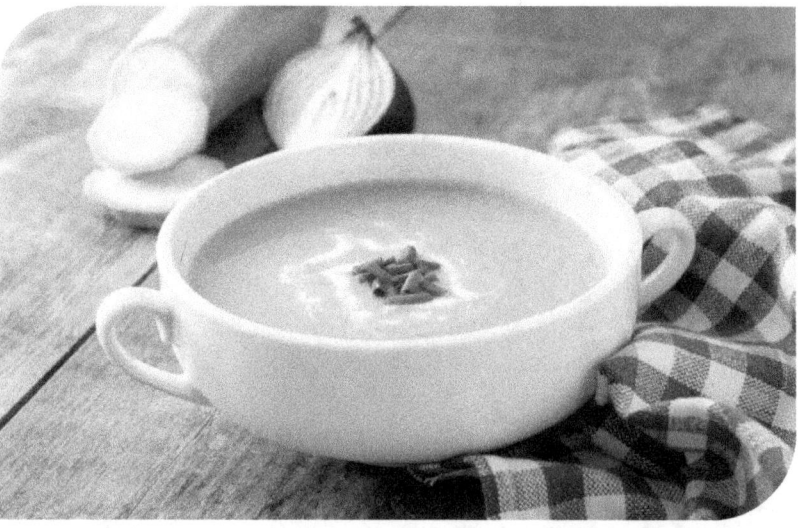

Ingredients

- 1 tablespoon of olive oil
- 1 medium onion
- 2 garlic cloves, minced
- 2 tbsp curry powder
- 1 large potato, peeled and chopped
- 2 medium zucchinis
- 4 cups low-sodium chicken stock
- ½ tablespoon of salt
- ¼ tbsp freshly ground black pepper

Steps to Cook

1. First of all, take a medium saucepan. Pour oil and put it to heat over medium heat.
2. Then add the onion. Cook it for about 7 or 8 minutes, stirring occasionally, but taking care that it does not stick to the bottom of the container.
3. Later, add the garlic to the saucepan, along with the curry powder and continue cooking and stirring, until they are directly attached to the onion, for which it should not take more than 1 minute per clock, in order to avoid the onion burns.
4. After that, add the remaining ingredients and heat them until they start to boil. Reduce the heat and allow approximately 20 minutes for the soup to be ready before turning off the heat and serving.

Nutritional Information:

- Calorie: 125
- Protein: 2.4g
- Fat: 10g
- Carbohydrates: 7.6g

Stewed Tofu

Servings: 2-4

Preparation time: 5 minutes

Cook time: 15 minutes

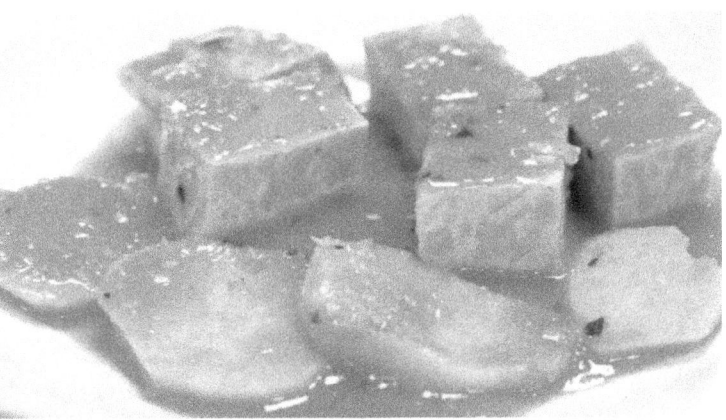

Ingredients

- ¼ lbs. by Tofu
- 2 small potatoes
- 1 onion
- Ketchup
- ½ glass of water
- Salt and parsley

Steps to Cook

1. Cut the onion finite and put it to sauté in the pan over low heat with a pinch of salt. Then add the fried tomato sauce, which you can substitute for crushed natural tomato. Let it on the fire for a couple of minutes and then add a little water and let a few more minutes. Afterwards pass everything through the mixer so that there was a uniform sauce, but you can leave it as is.
2. While the sauce was being made dice the tofu and prepare the potatoes in the microwave, make them in a steam case, without adding anything, just 5 minutes to the micro. If you prefer you can boil them normally.
3. Then put the tofu in the pot with a little oil to brown it and then add the sauce and finally the potatoes and let it cook over low heat for about 10 minutes. Correct salt and with a little parsley.

Nutritional Information:

- Calorie: 100
- Protein: 6g
- Fat: 6g
- Carbohydrates: 5g

Vegetable Stew

Servings: 2-4

Preparation time: 5 minutes

Cook time: 10-15 minutes

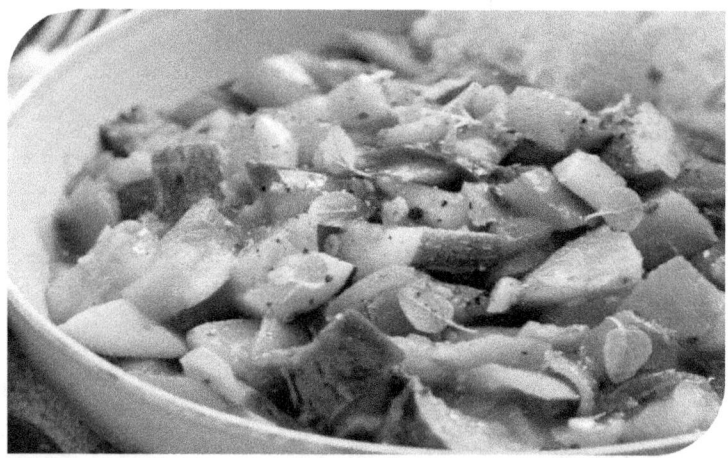

Ingredients

- A bunch of Swiss chard
- 2 cooked potatoes
- 2 cups baby carrots
- 2 cups artichokes
- 4 cloves of garlic
- 8 white asparagus
- 5 oz. of serrano ham in taquitos
- Extra virgin olive oil
- Salt

Steps to Cook

1. Peel the potato, cut it into cubes and cook it in water until tender.
2. Clean the chard, removing with the knife the ugliest parts, as well as the lower part of the stem and removing the outer layer.
3. Chop both the stem and the leaves, wash well and cook for 4 to 5 minutes, drain and reserve.
4. Cook the carrots about 8 minutes.
5. Once you have everything prepared, put a little extra virgin olive oil and some sliced garlic in the saucepan. When they start to brown, add everything and tide in for a few minutes. Finally, chop the asparagus and incorporate them, mix a little and your vegetable stew is ready to serve.

Nutritional Information:

- Calorie: 159
- Protein: 5.8g
- Fat: 3.8g
- Carbohydrates: 26g

Basque Porrusalda

Servings: 2

Preparation time: 5 minutes

Cook time: 20 minutes

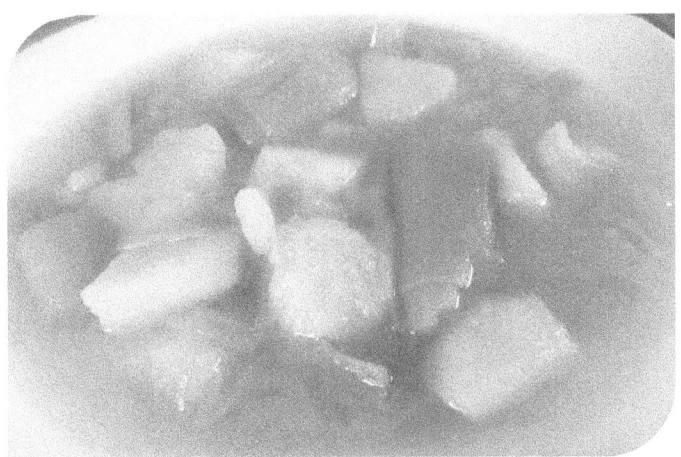

Ingredients

- 2 large leeks
- 4 medium potatoes
- Water
- salt and black pepper
- olive oil

Steps to Cook

1. We peel and clean the leek and the potato. Then cut them into large pieces
2. Pour a stream of olive oil in a high saucepan. Put it on medium-high heat and add the potato and the leek. Season with salt and pepper and cook for one minute, stirring constantly.
3. Pour water until it covers, approximately a finger or two above the vegetable.
4. Bring to a boil and let cook over medium heat for about 20 minutes. Until the vegetables are tender.

Nutritional Information:

- Calorie: 283.4
- Protein: 2.7g
- Fat: 20.5g
- Carbohydrates: 23.9g

Chapter 3
Salads

Vegan Mushroom And Tofu

Servings: 1

Preparation time: 5 minutes

Cook time: 15 minutes

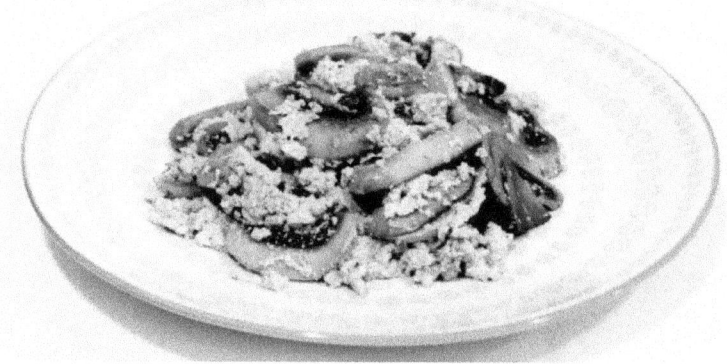

Ingredients

- 3 oz. of natural tofu
- 3 oz. fresh mushrooms
- 2 cloves of garlic
- 1 tablespoon soy sauce
- Extra virgin olive oil

Steps to Cook

1. Make your vegan scramble wash and laminate the mushrooms. Then peel and chop the garlic. Put it to sauté in a frying pan with a drizzle of extra virgin olive oil.
2. Move from time to time so that the mushrooms are taking color on both sides. Leave on medium heat until the mushrooms have reduced and start to brown.
3. Meanwhile, cut the chunk of tofu that you are going to use and crush it with a fork. Then add to the pan where you have the mushrooms and let them cook together for a couple of minutes. Finally add the soy sauce and stir well so that everything takes flavor.
4. If the sauce you use is not very salty, you can add a little salt to your vegan stir. Remove from the fire, let it temper a little.

Nutritional Information:

- Calorie: 150
- Protein: 5g
- Fat: 10g
- Carbohydrates: 9g

Quinoa Salad

Servings: 4

Preparation time: 10 minutes

Cook time: 15 minutes

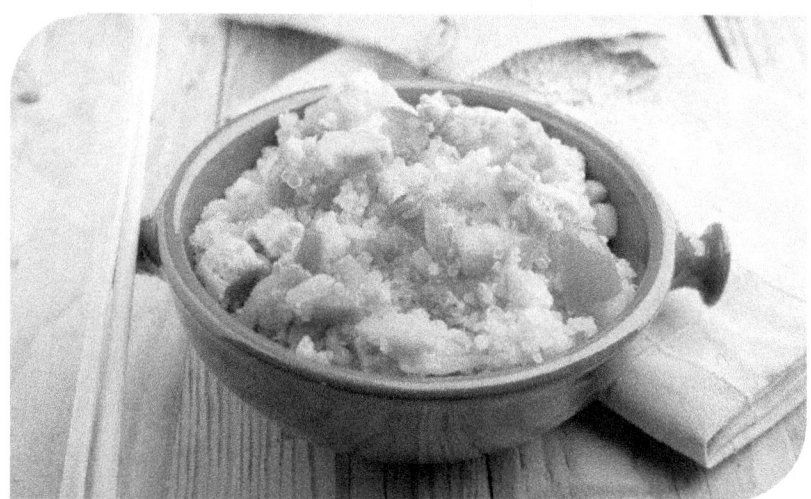

Ingredients

- 1 Cup of Quinoa
- 2 cups of vegetable broth
- 1 carrot
- ½ oz. Green cabbage
- Red cabbage 35 grams
- ½ oz. Red pepper
- 1 clove garlic
- Olive oil

Steps to Cook

1. Boil the broth
2. Add Quinoa over low heat for 20 minutes and stir.
3. Remove the Quinoa
4. Cut the red cabbage, the green and the pepper
5. Peel and cut the carrot into strips
6. Mix all the ingredients
7. Drizzle the salad with olive oil.

Nutritional Information:

- Calorie: 280
- Protein: 12g
- Fat: 9g
- Carbohydrates: 39g

Quinoa California Salad

Servings: 4

Preparation time: 10 minutes

Cook time: 10 minutes

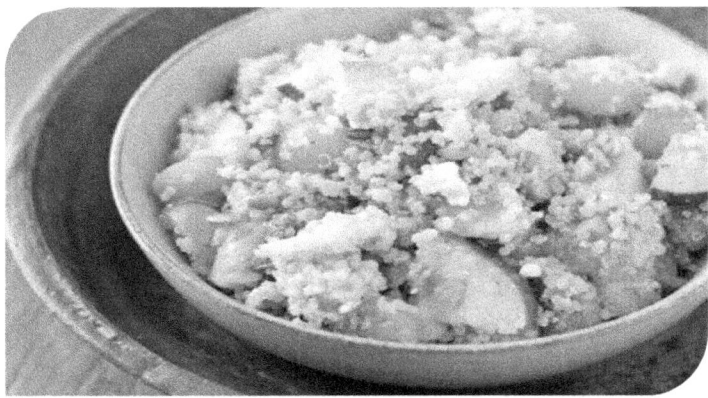

Ingredients

- 1 cup quinoa
- ¼ of Cup of balsamic vinegar
- Zest of 2 files
- 1 mango, peeled and diced
- 1 red bell pepper
- ½ cup edamame shells
- 1/3 cup red onion
- ¼ cup unsweetened coconut flakes
- ¼ cup sliced almonds
- ¼ cup raisins
- 2 tbsp chopped fresh coriander leaves

Steps to Cook

1. Put the quinoa to cook in a large pot with two cups of water, following the instructions on the package; then set it aside.
2. In a small bowl, beat the balsamic vinegar and the lemon zest; then put them aside
3. In a large bowl, combine the quinoa, mango, bell pepper, edamame, red onion, coconut flakes, almonds, raisins, and coriander. Pour the balsamic vinegar mixture on top of the salad and stir gently to combine.
4. Serve immediately.

Nutritional Information:

- Calorie: 280
- Protein: 12g
- Fat: 9g
- Carbohydrates: 39g

Greek Pasta Salad

Servings: 2

Preparation time: 5 minutes

Cooking time: 10-15 minutes

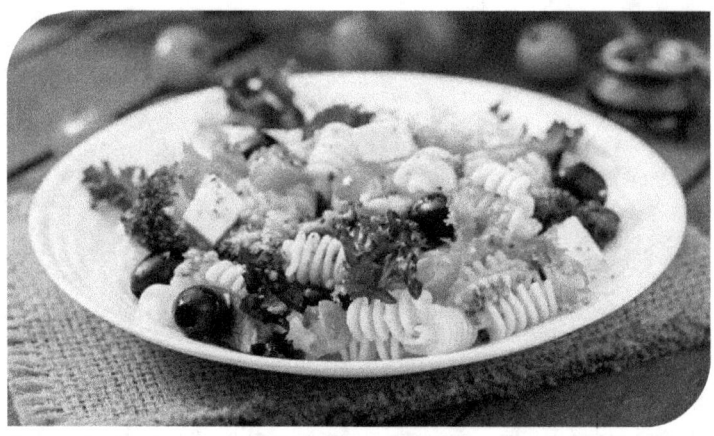

Ingredients

Vinaigrette:

- 4 tbsp of olive oil
- 2 tbsp of lemon juice
- 1 tbsp oregano
- 1 tbsp chopped mint
- Salt, pepper, to taste

Salad:

- ¼ lbs. of fusilli pasta
- 3 small cucumbers
- 18 cherry tomatoes
- ¼ lbs. of feta cheese
- 20 Greek olives
- ½ lbs. g artichoke hearts

Steps to Cook

1. For the vinaigrette, start by whisking all the ingredients mentioned in the list in a small bowl. Add additional lemon juice, olive oil, salt, and pepper to taste.
2. In a large pot bring water to a boil and add a tablespoon of salt. After a few minutes add the pasta to cook (make sure to follow the instructions on the back of the package). In case of opting for a quinoa paste, the estimated time is 9 minutes.
3. Drain the pasta and mix with the vinaigrette. When the pasta is cold add the cucumbers, tomatoes, olives, artichoke hearts, feta cheese and chives. Add another tablespoon of vinaigrette and serve on plates.

Nutritional Information:

- Calorie: 357
- Protein: 7.8g
- Fat: 20g
- Carbohydrates: 36g

Servings: 2

Thai Salad

Preparation time: 5 minutes

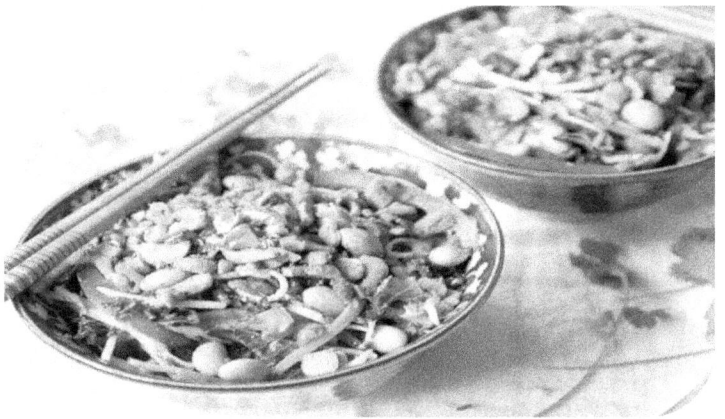

Ingredients

- 1 lb. clean zucchini
- 2 chopped chives
- 1 handful of unsalted roasted peanuts
- 2 garlic cloves, minced
- 15 g ginger, peeled and grated
- 3 tbsp soy sauce
- 2 tbsp of lime juice
- 1 good handful of Thai basil leaves
- 2 teaspoons of honey
- ½ chopped red chilli

Steps to Cook

1. Whisk the soy sauce, lime juice, honey, garlic, ginger, and white portion of the chives in a bowl.
2. Make spirals with the zucchini using the medium blade and reduce the size of the spaghetti.
3. Mix with the dressing and place in some bowls.
4. Top with basil, peanuts, chilli and green onions.

Nutritional Information:

- Calorie: 195
- Protein: 6.9g
- Fat: 8.8g
- Carbohydrates: 26g

Kale Salad With Chickpeas And Avocado

Servings: 2
Preparation time: 5 minutes

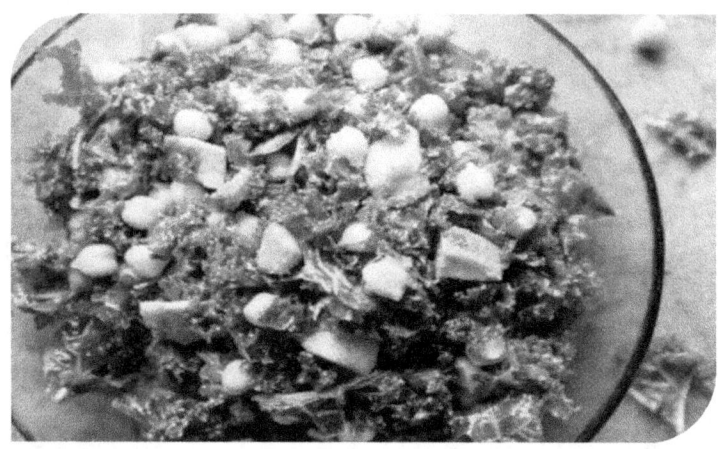

Ingredients

For the dressing:

- 2 tablespoons of lemon juice
- 1 clove garlic
- 1 teaspoon salt
- 2 teaspoon black pepper
- ¼ cup olive oil

For the salad:

- 5 cups kale
- ½ chickpea
- 1 ripe avocado

Steps to Cook

1. In a medium bowl, mix lemon juice, garlic, salt, and pepper, beat to combine.
2. Then, add the olive oil and beat until there is a creamy mixture.
3. Pour the previously prepared mixture onto the kale and gently stir the vinaigrette into the kale until all surfaces are coated and the kale has softened.
4. Add the chickpeas and avocado, cover and refrigerate until ready to serve, enjoy.

Nutritional Information:

- Calorie: 149
- Protein: 4g
- Fat: 8g
- Carbohydrates: 16g

Chickpea Salad With Avocado

Servings: 2

Preparation time: 5 minutes

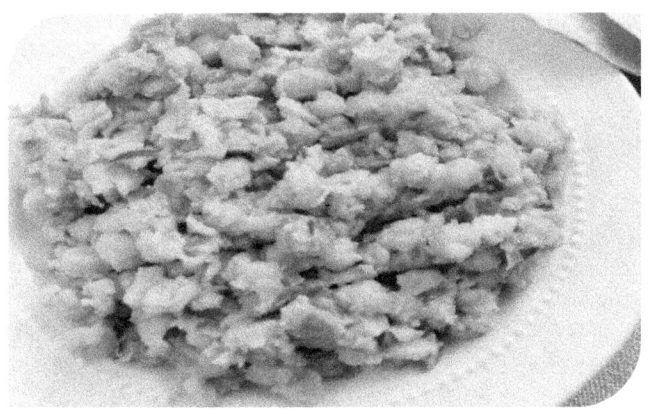

Ingredients

- 1 ½ cup cooked chickpeas
- 1 to mate red boy chopped into squares
- ¼ red purple onion, finely chopped
- 1 ripe boy avocado
- 1 lemon to taste
- Salt and pepper to taste
- Chopped cilantro
- Optional: olive oil to taste

Steps to Cook

1. Crush the cooked chickpeas with a bean masher or fork. Add the tomato, red onion and avocado. Crush again and mix well.
2. Season to taste with the lemon juice, salt and pepper. If you wish, you can add olive oil, herbs, paprika, garlic salt, fresh or pickled jalapeño pepper or whatever you prefer.
3. Serve alone, with toast, sandwich, crackers, or lettuce leaves to make chickpea taquitos.

Nutritional Information:

- Calorie: 149
- Protein: 4g
- Fat: 8g
- Carbohydrates: 16g

Lentil Salad

Servings: 1
Preparation time: 5 minutes

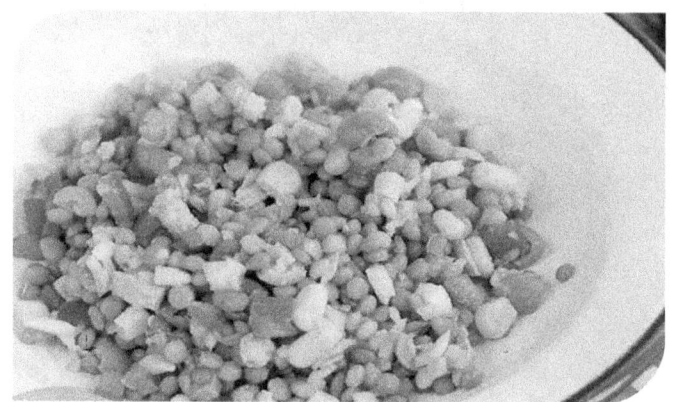

Ingredients

- 1 lbs. lentils, preserved.
- 1 red pepper
- 1 chive
- Pitted olives
- Sweet corn
- Apple vinegar
- Salt
- Extra virgin olive oil

Steps to Cook

1. Take the lentils out of the jar and wash them well under a cold running tap.
2. Drain them well, put in a bowl and add the bell pepper, chives and olives, all finely chopped.
3. Add the corn a pinch of salt, apple cider vinegar and extra virgin olive oil to taste.
4. Store in the fridge until serving time and enjoy this healthy and simple lentil salad!

Nutritional Information:

- Calorie: 255
- Protein: 12g
- Fat: 10g
- Carbohydrates: 31g

Perfect Summer Pasta Salad

Servings: 2
Preparation time: 5 minutes
Cooking time: 10-15 minutes

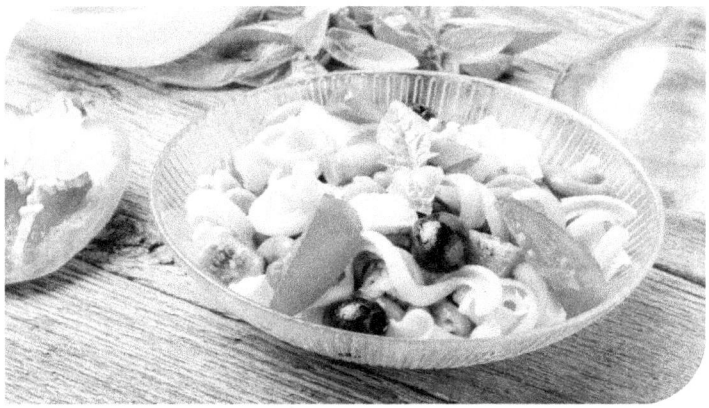

Ingredients

- A quarter of a packet of dry, uncooked ringlet noodles
- 1 ripe tomato
- 10 green or black olives
- 1 ripe avocado
- 1 coriander sprig
- Roasted sunflower seeds
- Olive oil
- Aceto
- Honey
- Pepper

Steps to Cook

1. Peel the avocado, remove the pit and cut it into medium cubes. Wash the tomato and cut it into cubes the same size as the avocado. On the other hand, cut the olives into thin slices and throw the pit. Wash the coriander, remove the stems and chop it very small.
2. In a saucepan with water, salt and a stream of oil, cook the ringlet noodles. Water and noodles should always be calculated in equal amounts. Once the noodles are strained and cold, add a dash of oil to them so they do not stick and place all the ingredients in a salad bowl.
3. Top with roasted sunflower seeds, and season with olive oil, salt and pepper. To give it a gourmet touch you can add a teaspoon of honey.

Nutritional Information:

- Calorie: 357
- Protein: 7.8g
- Fat: 20g
- Carbohydrates: 36g

Asparagus Salad With Blueberries And Vinaigrette

Servings: 2
Preparation time: 5 minutes
Cooking time: 5-10 minutes

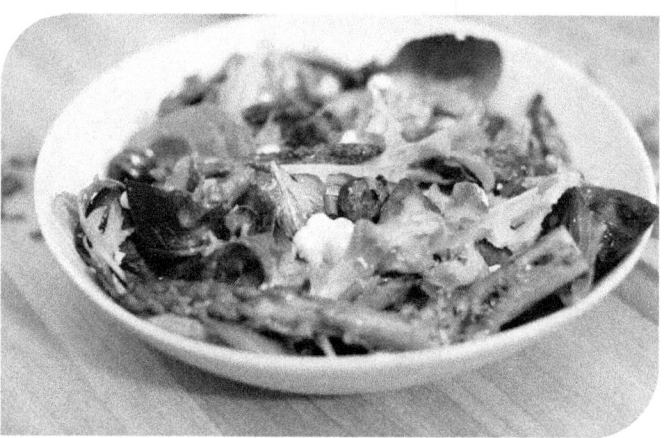

Ingredients

- 20 clean asparagus
- 4 shallots filleted
- 2 tablespoons olive oil
- 1 cup blueberries

For the vinaigrette:

- ¼ cup balsamic vinegar
- 1 tbsp Dijon mustard
- 1 tbsp Honey Bee
- ½ cup olive oil
- Salt and pepper
- 1 cup peppermint leaf
- 3 oz. roasted and chopped hazelnuts

Steps to Cook

For the vinaigrette:

1. Cut the asparagus into thirds.
2. Blanch and place in a bowl with water and ice to stop cooking. Drain and reserve.
3. Mix the vinegar with the mustard and pour the olive oil a little bit until it is integrated.
4. Season with salt and pepper and add honey. Mixture.

For the salad:

5. Mix the asparagus with the shallot and blueberries. Bathe with the vinaigrette and mix.
6. Serve and sprinkle with hazelnuts. Decorate with fresh mint leaves.

Nutritional Information:

- Calorie: 69
- Protein: 3.6g
- Fat: 0.8g
- Carbohydrates: 15.1g

Kale Salad

Servings: 2-4
Preparation time: 5 minutes

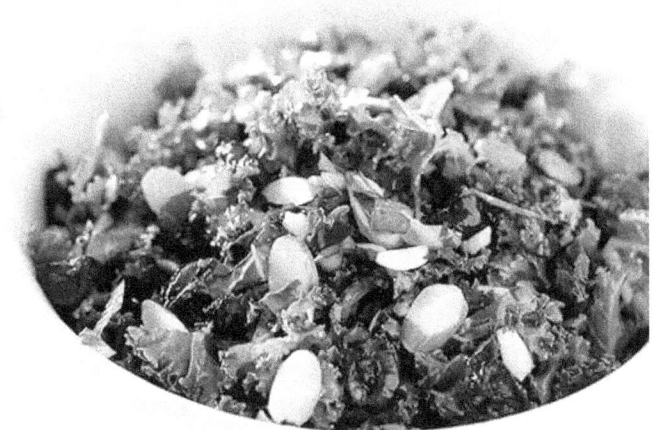

Ingredients

- 2 Kale leaves or kale
- 1 sweet potato or sweet potato
- ½ bell pepper or red pepper
- ½ zucchini
- Alfalfa sprouts

Steps to Cook

1. Peel the sweet potato, cut it into slices and steam it next to the red pepper.
2. Grate the zucchini.
3. To assemble the salad, place the kale leaves in a bowl and on them the sweet potato, the pepper cut into strips, the zucchini and sprinkle with the alfalfa sprouts.
4. Season with sesame or olive oil, salt, pepper and spices to taste.

Nutritional Information:

- Calorie: 84
- Protein: 1.2g
- Fat: 7.3g
- Carbohydrates: 3.9g

Chapter 4

Pasta & Noodles

Vegan Noodles

Servings: 1
Preparation time: 5 minutes
Cook time: 15-20 minutes

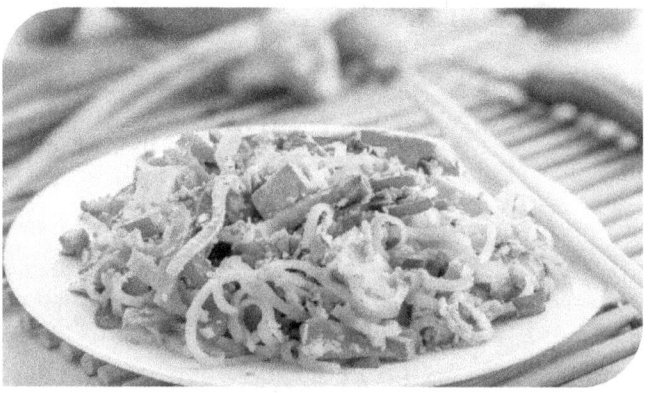

Ingredients

- Vegetables: peppers green, red and yellow, zucchini and carrot.
- Vegan noodles
- Vegetables soup
- Soy sauce
- Salt and oil

Steps to Cook

1. Clean the vegetables well and cut them into strips.
2. In a non-stick pot, heat the oil and add the vegetables except the zucchini. Let them simmer, when they start to take color add the zucchini and shortly after add the vegetable stock that you have previously heated. No need to pour too much, loosely covering the vegetables.
3. Then put soy sauce to taste, stir and when you see that the broth is boiling well, add the noodles. Let it cook for about 5 minutes. Remove from the fire, to rest a few minutes and that's it!

Nutritional Information:

- Calorie: 174
- Protein: 6g
- Fat: 3g
- Carbohydrates: 34g

Zucchini Pasta

Servings: 2
Preparation time: 5 minutes
Cook time: 5-10 minutes

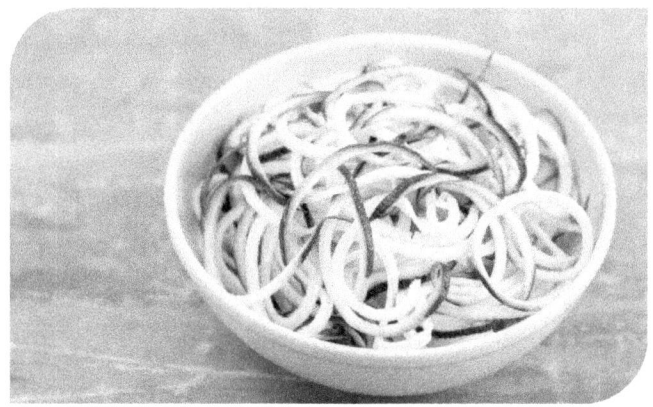

Ingredients

- 1 zucchini
- 2 garlic cloves, crushed
- 2 teaspoons of olive oil
- Salt
- Black pepper
- 2 tablespoons of water
- Grated Parmesan cheese

Steps to Cook

1. Cut the zucchini into long ribbons, using a mandolin or a knife. Cut the ribbon lengthwise, so that fettucinis are left as strands.
2. Heat a skillet over medium-high heat until hot. Add 1 teaspoon of oil and the crushed garlic. Add the zucchini strands and stir. Add Italian seasoning, salt and black pepper to taste. Add 2 tablespoons of water and stir a couple of minutes or until the zucchini is "al dente".
3. Remove to a plate with grated Parmesan cheese and serve.

Nutritional Information:

- Calorie: 20
- Protein: 1.4g
- Fat: 0.4g
- Carbohydrates: 3.7g

Asian Spaghetti With Peanut Butter And Chilli

Servings: 6
Preparation time: 5 minutes
Cook time: 15-20 minutes

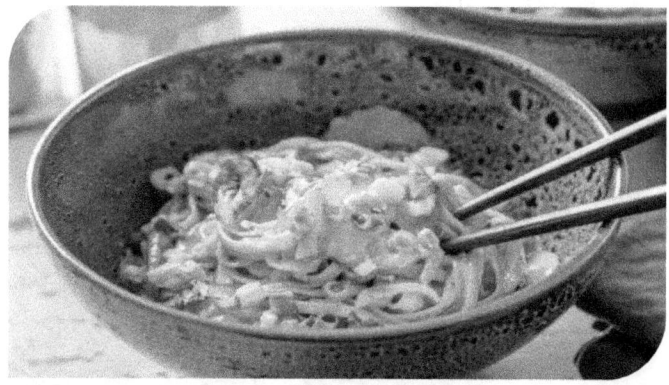

Ingredients

- 1-pound dried noodles
- 1/8 cup sesame oil
- ¼ cup soy sauce
- ½ - 1 tbsp of sweetener
- 1 ½ tsp vinegar
- 2 teaspoons of salt
- 1 cup chopped fresh coriander
- 4-8 green chives
- 1-3 tbsp spicy red chili sauce
- 3 tbsp of peanut butter
- 2 tbsp coconut cream
- Peanuts (optional)

Steps to Cook

1. Bring the noodles or spaghetti to a boil in a saucepan with salt water until "al dente". Usually 12-15 minutes. Follow package directions.
2. While cooking, prepare the sauce:
3. Combine sesame oil, soy sauce, sweetener, vinegar, salt, chili sauce, coconut, and peanut butter.
4. Drain the noodles or spaghetti when done.
5. Stir in the sauce, and add the coriander and green chives.
6. They can be served cold or hot.
7. Add the peanuts and chives.

Nutritional Information:

- Calorie: 330
- Protein: 12g
- Fat: 5g
- Carbohydrates: 60g

Pasta To Orange With Soybean

Servings: 1
Preparation time: 5 minutes
Cook time: 10-15 minutes

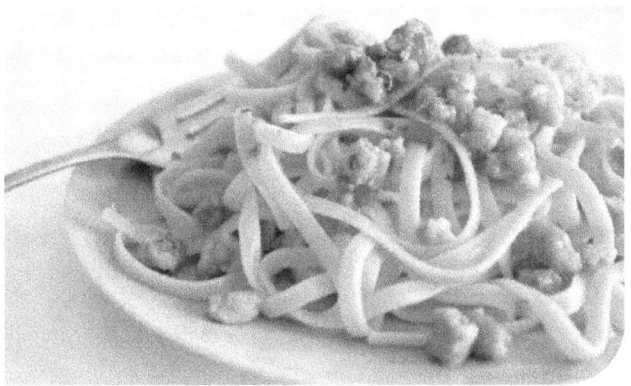

Ingredients

- Pasta with orange
- 1 cup of textured soy.
- The juice of an orange.
- 1 tbsp of white wine.
- 1 tbsp of apple cider vinegar
- 1 tbsp soy margarine
- ½ tablet of vegetable broth

Steps to Cook

1. Bring the water to boil for the pasta, add a little salt. While it starts to boil, soak the soybeans and squeeze the orange. When the water starts to boil, put the pasta until it is ready. Then drain and ready.
2. **For the sauce**:
3. melt the tablespoon of margarine in a frying pan and when it is liquid add the orange juice and let it boil for a couple of minutes, then add the wine and vinegar and finally the half broth tablet, to be able to be already diluted in a couple of teaspoons of the own broth that you are preparing so that there are no lumps later. Let it boil for a minute or so and add the soy. Let the broth decrease and the soy absorbs it almost completely. Remove from heat. Put some parsley and serve.

Nutritional Information:

- Calorie: 174
- Protein: 6g
- Fat: 3g
- Carbohydrates: 34g

Pasta With Almond Cream, Red Pepper And Basil

Servings: 4
Preparation time: 5 minutes
Cooking time: 30 minutes

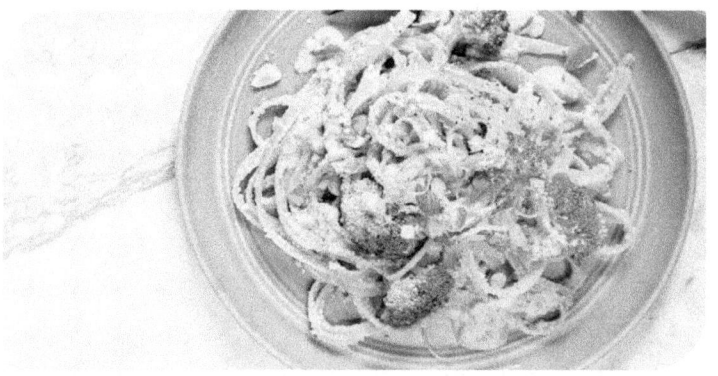

Ingredients

- 3 oz. tomato sauce
- 2 small roasted red peppers
- 1 ½ oz. Ecomil almond cream
- ¼ tablespoon dried oregano
- salt and pepper to taste
- 100g of pasta

Steps to Cook

1. Mix the tomato sauce, the peppers, the almond cream, the oregano and salt and pepper.
2. Cook the pasta and cover with the sauce.
3. Garnish with fresh basil and nutritional yeast and enjoy!

Nutritional Information:

- Calorie: 192
- Protein: 6.9g
- Fat: 10.5g
- Carbohydrates: 15.5g

Pasta To Pesto With Bimi

Servings: 2-4
Preparation time: 15 minutes
Cook time: 20-25 minutes

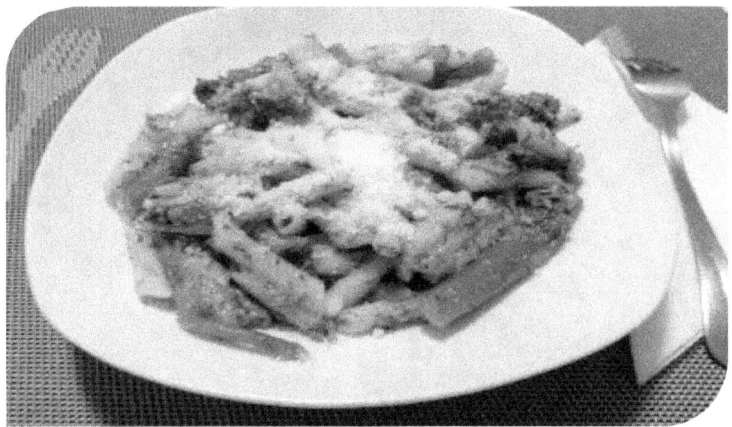

Ingredients

- 8 stalks of Bimi
- 4 tsp fresh basil
- 4 tsp fresh spinach
- 6 tsp raw almonds
- 1 clove garlic
- ¼ tsp extra virgin olive oil
- 1 tablespoon nutritional yeast
- ½ lbs. pasta
- Salt and pepper

Steps to Cook

Prepare the pesto:
1. Add the basil, spinach, almonds, garlic, oil, nutritional yeast and a pinch of salt. Crush until a more or less homogeneous paste is left. If you see that you like it a little lighter you can add a little more oil to make it less thick.
2. On the other hand, bring the pasta to a boil. When the pasta is almost done, prepare the bimi grilled. If you have not tried it, it is a mixture between broccoli and a type of oriental cabbage, kai-lán. It only takes about 3-4 minutes to make in the pan. Put a little olive oil and then salt and pepper, and if you have, a little garlic powder.
3. To present it, with the pasta and pesto already mixed or leaving the pesto simply on top and each one mixing it in the dish itself.

Nutritional Information:

- Calorie: 160
- Protein: 4g
- Fat: 7g
- Carbohydrates: 18g

Pasta With Mushrooms And Tofu Sauce

Servings: 2
Preparation time: 5 minutes
Cook time: 15-20 minutes

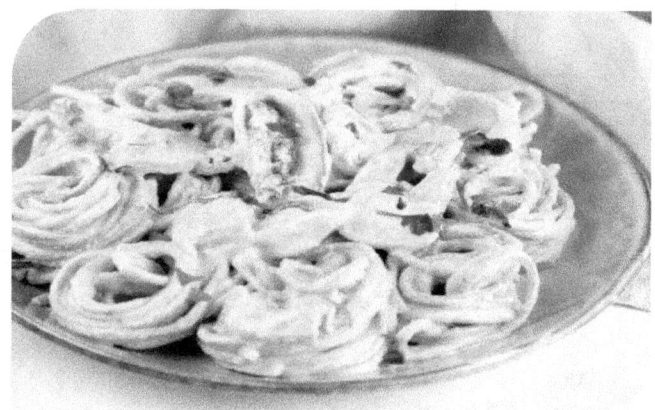

Ingredients

- 1 lbs. mushrooms
- ½ lbs. tofu
- 1 cup soy milk
- ½ cup of water
- 3 oz. whole wheat spaghetti
- 1 splash of white wine
- Salt
- Pepper
- Parsley

Steps to Cook

1. Wash and cut the mushrooms into slices. Put it in the pan with a splash of olive oil and salt. Let them cook until they are usually in the water, reduce their size and remain slightly golden.
2. On the other hand, put the whole pasta to cook in water.
3. Meanwhile, put diced tofu, milk and water in mixing glass. Crush until you have a homogeneous cream.
4. Add to the pan with the mushrooms, stir and add a little salt, pepper to taste and a splash of white wine.
5. Let it all together for about 5 minutes. Drain the pasta and also add it to the pan, stirring so that all the pasta is impregnated with sauce.
6. Put some fresh parsley and eat!

Nutritional Information:

- Calorie: 333.5
- Protein: 616.1g
- Fat: 7.9g
- Carbohydrates: 51.7g

Ramen

Servings: 4
Preparation time: 5 minutes
Cook time: 25 minutes

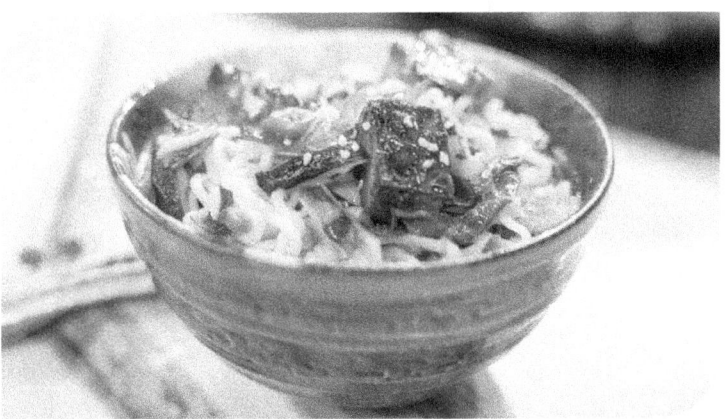

Ingredients

- 6 packages of ramen noodles
- 10 tbsp low-salt soy sauce
- 3 garlic cloves
- 2 tbsp minced ginger
- 3 tbsp of sesame oil
- 7 cups of vegetable broth
- 3 tbsp of sake (Japanese wine)
- 1 tablespoon of salt
- 3 spoonsful of sugar

Steps to Cook

1. Heat the sesame oil in a saucepan. Chop the garlic and brown them in the oil along with the minced ginger. When this mixture is lightly browned, add the broth and wait for it to boil.
2. When it boils, add the sugar, soy sauce, sake, and salt. Boil for 5 minutes, add the noodles and wait for them to cook, about 5 minutes.
3. Serve the soup. You can add boiled egg, breaded chicken, and nori seaweed to complement the ramen.

Nutritional Information:

- Calorie: 188
- Protein: 5g
- Fat: 7g
- Carbohydrates: 27g

Noodles With Tofu And Peanut Dressing

Servings: 4
Preparation time: 5 minutes
Cooking time: 30 minutes

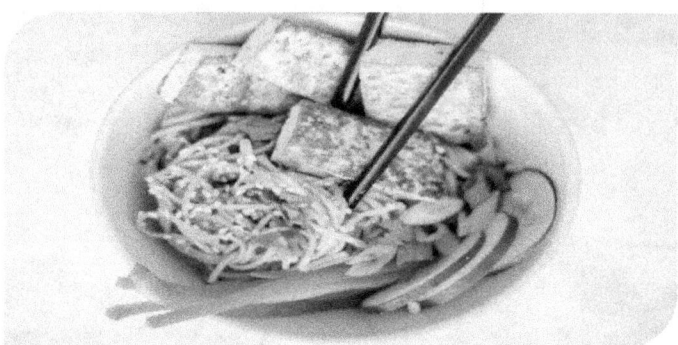

Ingredients

For the dressing:
- 1 garlic
- 2 tbsp sesame oil
- 3 tbsp peanut butter
- 2 tsp grated ginger
- 3 tbsp lemon juice
- 2 tbsp soy sauce
- 2 tsp brown sugar

For the noodles:
- 340 g extra firm tofu
- 170 g soba noodles
- ½ tablespoon olive oil
- 1 small red pepper
- ½ cucumber
- 1 carrot
- 4 onions
- ¼ cup coriander, finely chopped

Steps to Cook

For the dressing:
1. In a blender, place the garlic, sesame oil, peanut butter, grated ginger, lemon juice, soy sauce and brown sugar. Blend until obtaining a homogeneous mixture.

For the noodles:
2. Place a plate of heavy material on top of the tofu. Leave squeezing 30 minutes, so that the greatest amount of liquid comes out. Cut the tofu into small cubes. Heat a non-stick frying pan, without oil, fry the tofu cubes until golden brown on both sides.
3. Cook the noodles according to the directions on the package. Drain and soak in cold water. Transfer the noodles to a large bowl and mix them with the olive oil, this prevents them from sticking.
4. Julienne the cucumber, cucumber, and carrots. Cut the onions into slices.
5. Combine the vegetables with the noodles. Add the dressing and mix to integrate completely. Add the tofu squares and mix. Test and season if necessary.

Nutritional Information:

- Calorie: 429
- Protein: 19g
- Fat: 18g
- Carbohydrates: 49g

Pasta With Vegan Pesto

Servings: 4
Preparation time: 10 minutes
Cooking time: 10 minutes

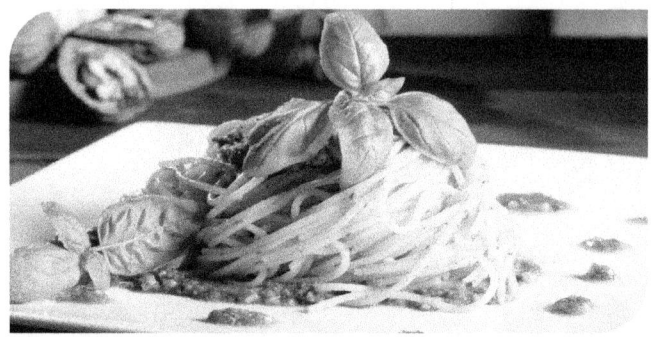

Ingredients

- 1 bunch of basil
- ¾ cup cashews or walnuts.
- ¼ cup olive oil
- 2 cloves of garlic
- 2 tablespoons nutritional yeast
- 2 tablespoons of lemon juice
- ¼ teaspoon of salt
- Ground pepper
- 1 lb. of dry pasta

Steps to Cook

1. In a large pot of water, boil the pasta.
2. Peel the garlic, and squeeze lemon juice.
3. Mix everything (basil, cashews, olive oil, garlic, nutritional yeast, lemon juice, salt, and pepper) in a food processor. Just until everything is ground into a paste, but retains a bit of texture.
4. When the pasta is cooked, drain and then put it back in the pot. Add the pesto to the pot with the pasta and stir until well combined. Serve immediately.

Nutritional Information:

- Calorie: 160
- Protein: 4g
- Fat: 7g
- Carbohydrates: 18g

Pasta With Avocado Cream

Servings: 3
Preparation time: 5 minutes
Cooking time: 20 minutes

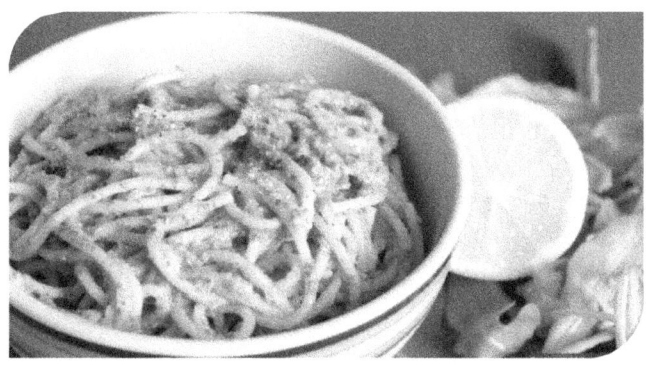

Ingredients

- 12 oz of spaghetti
- 2 ripe avocados, shelled and seedless
- ½ cup fresh basil leaves
- 2 cloves of garlic
- 2 tbsp of freshly squeezed lemon juice
- Salt and pepper to taste
- Olive oil
- ½ cup cherry tomatoes, cut in half

Steps to Cook

1. In a large pot of boiling salted water, cook the pasta according to the package directions.
2. While this is the pasta we will make the avocado cream, combine the avocados, the basil, the garlic and the lemon juice in the food processor; season with salt and pepper to taste. With the engine running, add a stream of olive oil until smooth; Reserve.
3. In a large bowl, combine the pasta, avocado sauce, and cherry tomatoes.
4. Serve immediately.

Nutritional Information:

- Calorie: 445.1
- Protein: 9.5g
- Fat: 28.1g
- Carbohydrates: 46.7g

Pasta With Cheese Mix

Servings: 2
Preparation time: 10 minutes
Cook time: 12-15 minutes

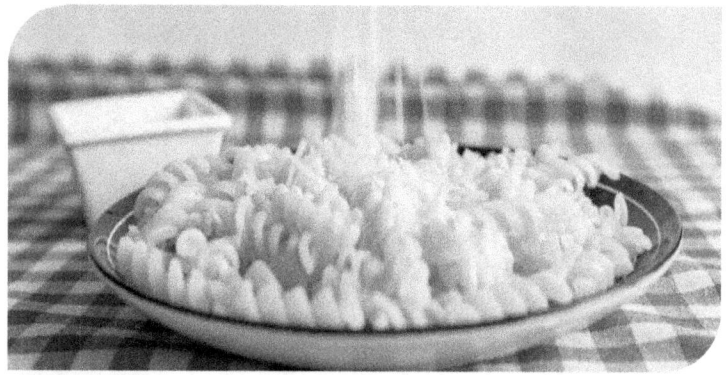

Ingredients

- 1 tbsp. butter
- 2 cups cooked noodles.
- 1 cup of mozzarella
- 1 cup shredded cheddar
- 3 tbsp. milk
- ¼ cup of tomatoes
- Chopped parsley
- 2 tbsp. grated parmesan
- salt pepper

Steps to Cook

1. Butter an oven safe skillet.
2. Pour the previously cooked pasta into the pan, adding part of the mozzarella and the grated cheddar.
3. Add the tablespoons of milk, the crushed tomatoes and finish with more cheese
4. Sprinkle with parsley and Parmesan.
5. Take to gratin for 12/15m in oven at 400°F.

Nutritional Information:

- Calorie: 250
- Protein: 6g
- Fat: 1g
- Carbohydrates: 54g

Chapter 5

Rice & Grains

Granola, Greek Yogurt And Red Berries

Servings: 1
Preparation time: 2 minutes
Cooking: 15-20 minutes

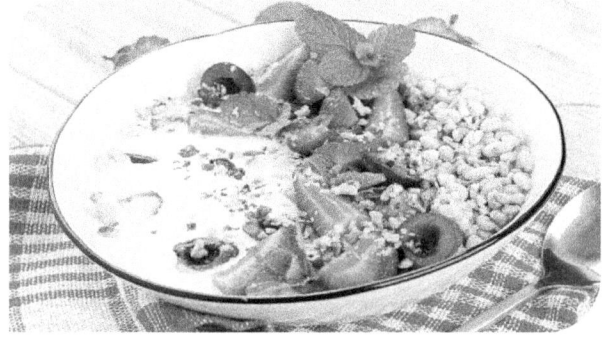

Ingredients

- 3 or 4 tbsp of granola
- 1 Greek yogurt
- 2 tbsp of red berries

Steps to Cook

For the granola:

1. Mix all ingredients in a bowl
2. Spread the mixture on a cookie sheet
3. Bake for 15-20 minutes at 180°C
4. While it is in the oven, stir it so that the whole mixture is browned equally
5. Add the granola in the glass or bowl where you are going to eat.
6. And add the yogurt and red berries.

Nutritional Information:

- Calorie: 250.9
- Protein: 14g
- Fat: 7g
- Carbohydrates: 34g

Integral Rice With Pineapple And Coconut

Servings: 2
Preparation time: 30 minutes
Cooking time: 40-50 minutes

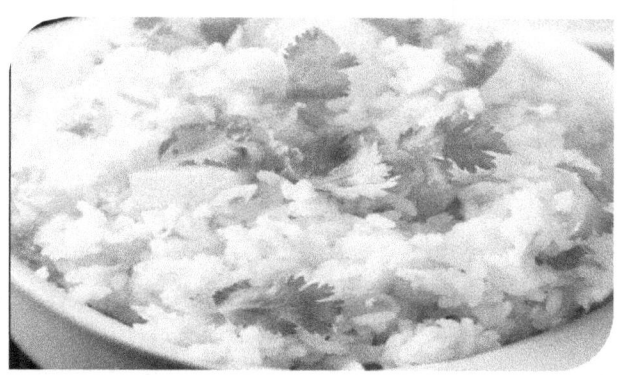

Ingredients

- 1 cup brown rice
- 1 ½ oz. of sliced almonds
- 1 tablespoon of coconut oil
- 2 ½ cups hot water
- 1 pinch of salt
- 5 pineapple slices in squares
- ½ fresh coconut, broken and filleted

Steps to Cook

1. Rinse the rice and let it soak for 30 minutes.
2. Meanwhile sauté the almonds in a skillet to brown, reserve a moment.
3. Drain the rice. Place it in a pan with the coconut oil to lightly brown. Add the water and, when it starts to boil, add the salt. Cover the saucepan and reduce the heat. Continue until the water is consumed.
4. Serve the rice in bowls, add the pineapple, coconut and almonds.

Nutritional Information:

- Calorie: 187.6
- Protein: 3.1g
- Fat: 5.2g
- Carbohydrates: 32g

Almond And Coconut Granola

Servings: 4
Preparation time: 5 minutes
Cooking time: 25 minutes

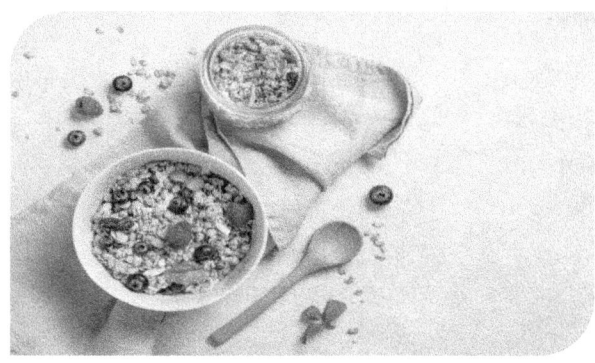

Ingredients

- 1 cup rolled oats
- ¼ cup grated coconut
- ¼ cup chopped almonds
- ¼ cup amaranth
- ¼ cup agave honey
- 1 ½ tablespoons of coconut oil
- ½ tbsp of vanilla extract
- ¼ tbsp cinnamon

Steps to Cook

1. Mix all the ingredients in a bowl. When they are well mixed, place the mixture on a baking sheet.
2. Preheat oven to 350 ° F for 15 minutes. Bake at 350 ° F for 20-25 minutes.
3. Remove the mixture from the oven and let cool for 1 hour. Reserve in a hermetically sealed container for up to 10 days.

Nutritional Information:

- Calorie: 270.1
- Protein: 6g
- Fat: 14g
- Carbohydrates: 32g

Mango And Peach Smoothie Bowl

Servings: 4
Preparation time: 5 minutes
Cooking time: 5 minutes

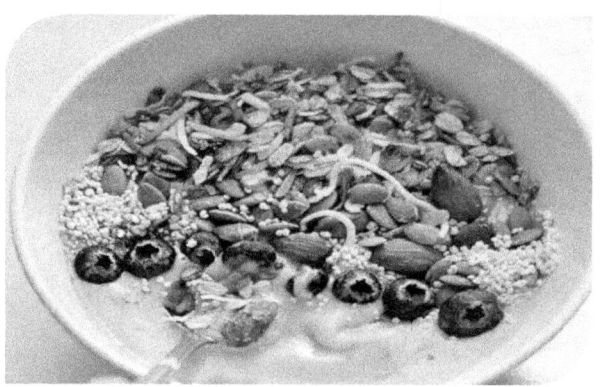

Ingredients

For the smoothie:
- 1 ripe peach, chopped
- 1 ripe mango, chopped
- 1 ripe banana, chopped
- ¼ cup coconut milk

To serve:
- ½ cup granola
- ¼ cup amaranth
- 2 tablespoons of pumpkin seeds
- ¼ cup blueberries

Steps to Cook

1. Place all the ingredients for the smoothie in a food processor or blender capable of crushing ice. Press until all the ingredients are perfectly incorporated.
2. Serve in bowls and decorate to your liking.

Nutritional Information:

- Calorie: 352
- Protein: 23.4g
- Fat: 9.3g
- Carbohydrates: 46.4g

Organic Quinoa

Servings: 4
Preparation time: 5 minutes
Cook time: 15-20 minutes

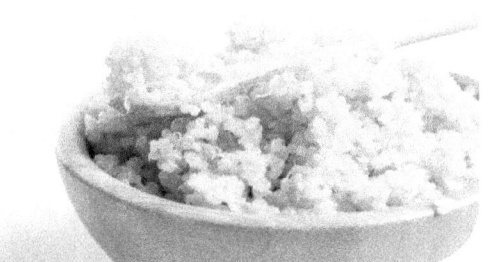

Ingredients

- 1 cup organic quinoa
- 2 cups of water
- ½ teaspoon of salt

Steps to Cook

1. Rinse the quinoa in a fine strainer until the water runs clear.
2. Drain and transfer to a medium saucepan.
3. Add the water and salt and bring to a boil.
4. Cover, reduce the heat to medium-low and simmer until the water is absorbed, (about 15 to 20 minutes).
5. Set it aside off the heat for 5 minutes; uncover and remove the lint with a fork.

Nutritional Information:

- Calorie: 120
- Protein: 4.4g
- Fat: 1.9g
- Carbohydrates: 21.3g

Quinoa With Boricua Flavor

Servings: 4
Preparation time: 5 minutes
Cook time: 20-25 minutes

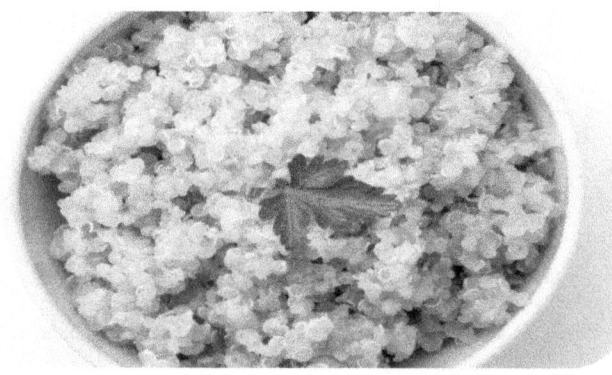

Ingredients

- 1 cup Quinoa
- 2 teaspoons canola oil
- Half medium chopped onion
- 2 garlic cloves, minced
- 14 ounces vegetable broth
- ¼ cup chopped almonds
- 3/4 cup chopped fresh coriander
- ½ cup chopped chives
- 2 tablespoons of lemon juice
- ¼ teaspoon of salt

Steps to Cook

1. Put the toasted Quinoa in a large dry skillet over medium heat. Stir frequently until crisp and aromatic.
2. Pass through a fine strainer and rinse well.
3. Heat the oil over medium heat in a large saucepan. Add a square (two tablespoons) of Puerto Rican sofrito, the onion and cook, stirring frequently, until smooth (2 to 3 minutes).
4. Add garlic and cook, stirring, for 30 seconds. Add Quinoa and broth and cook.
5. Reduce heat, cover and cook until Quinoa is smooth and most of the liquid has been absorbed (20 to 25 minutes).
6. Add to the Quinoa, the flaked almonds, the coriander, the chives, the lemon juice and the salt, mix gently with a fork.

Nutritional Information:

- Calorie: 120
- Protein: 4.4g
- Fat: 1.9g
- Carbohydrates: 21.3g

Instant Couscous

Servings: 4
Preparation time: 10 minutes
Cook time: 10-15 minutes

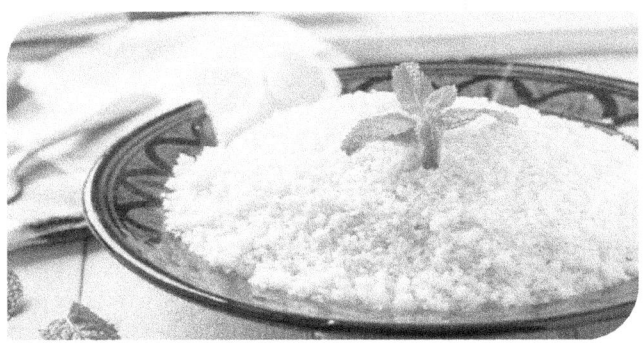

Ingredients

- 1 cup of water (or better low-sodium vegetable broth).
- 1 cup of couscous.
- 1-2 teaspoons of olive oil.
- A little salt according to your taste and preference.

Steps to Cook

1. Fill a medium saucepan with the water or vegetable stock.
2. Add the olive oil and salt.
3. Bring the water to a boil.
4. Add the couscous and turn off the heat. Stir to moisten, cover, and wait 10 minutes.
5. If it has not absorbed all the water, let it rest for a few more minutes.
6. Serve it with beans, chickpeas, or sauces and salad.

Nutritional Information:

- Calorie: 150
- Protein: 5g
- Fat: 0g
- Carbohydrates: 30g

Rice, Beans And Kale With Dressing

Servings: 4
Preparation time: 10 minutes
Cooking time: 40-45 minutes

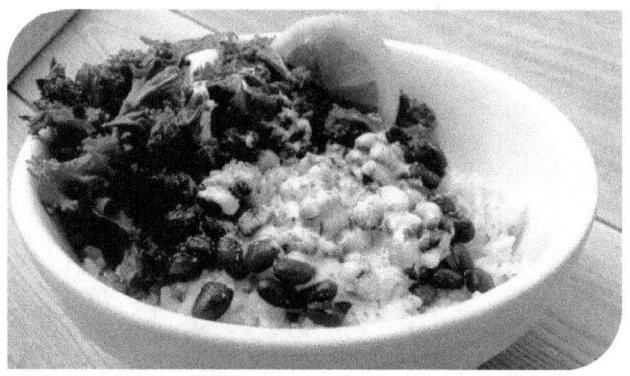

Ingredients

- 1 can of black beans
- 1 cup of tahini or hummus
- ½ cup lemon juice
- 1 tbsp. fresh dill
- 1 cup cooked brown rice
- 1 bunch of steamed kale
- 1 tsp. vegan parmesan (optional)

Steps to Cook

1. Heat the black beans in a medium saucepan over medium heat.
2. Mix the tahini, lemon juice, and dill in a small bowl until the consistency resembles a dressing.
3. Place a layer of the cooked brown rice, black beans, and kale in the bowl and top with the tahini dressing.
4. Sprinkle with vegan parmesan cheese and enjoy!

Nutritional Information:

- Calorie: 497.1
- Protein: 20.9g
- Fat: 15.3g
- Carbohydrates: 70.8g

Risotto Of Quinoa

Servings: 2
Preparation time: 5 minutes
Cooking time: 20 minutes

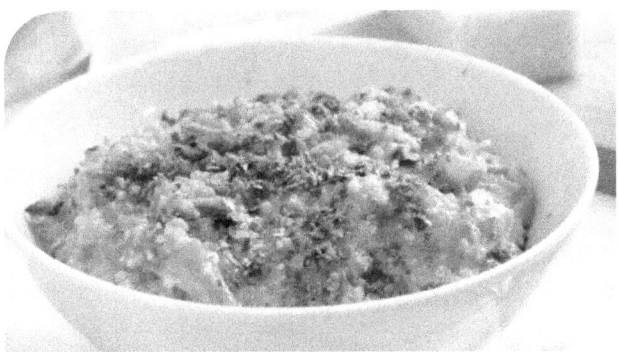

Ingredients

- 1 cup quinoa
- 1 cup of mushrooms
- 1 scallion
- 1 zucchini
- 2 cups of water
- thyme
- Parmesan
- nutmeg

Steps to Cook

1. Let the quinoa soak for at least 1 hour, then rinse it and cook it in 2 cups of water over low heat until the quinoa absorbs all the water.
2. Meanwhile, in a frying pan add a splash of oil and sauté the previously cut mushrooms in slices, the zucchini cut into slices, the finely chopped chives and a sprig of thyme, salt and pepper to taste.
3. In a bowl add the quinoa, the vegetables, the nutmeg and stir, sprinkle over the grated Parmesan cheese.

Nutritional Information:

- Calorie: 221.4
- Protein: 8.3g
- Fat: 2.9g
- Carbohydrates: 34.6g

Rice With Lentils

Servings: 3
Preparation time: 5 minutes
Cooking time: 50-60 minutes

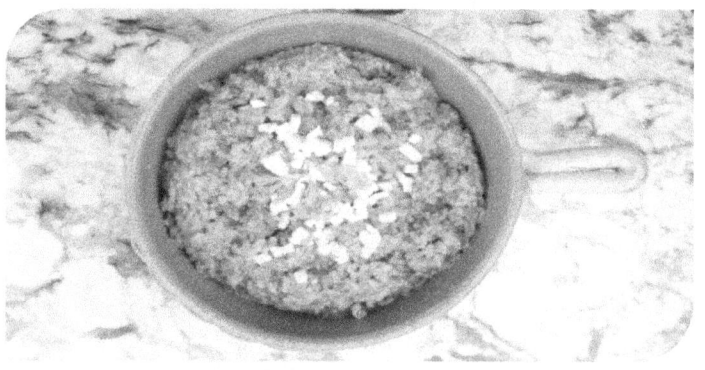

Ingredients

- 1 lbs. of lentils washed
- 1 bell pepper
- 1 red onion, chopped
- 1 chopped tomato
- 3 cup rice
- 1 tbsp butter
- Cumin
- Salt
- paprika
- Olive oil to taste

Steps to Cook

1. Make a rehash with the onion, pepper, and tomatoes.
2. Put paprika to taste as well as salt, cumin and oil.
3. When it is already fried add 3 cups of water when it starts to boil put the lentils ... when you see that the lentils
4. They are soft put the rice and rectify salt ... let cook until it bursts.
5. After it has burst you can put 1 tablespoon of butter.
6. Ready to serve!

Nutritional Information:

- Calorie: 140
- Protein: 12g
- Fat: 0.5g
- Carbohydrates: 23g

Choclo Grill

Servings: 4
Preparation time: 3 minutes
Cook time: 10 minutes

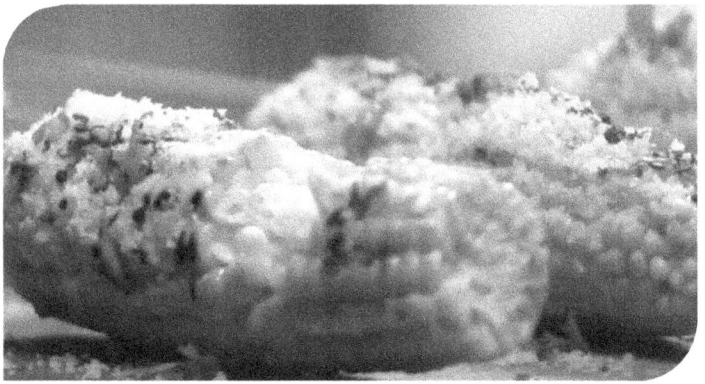

Ingredients

- 4 corn
- chile spicy
- 200 g of butter
- 300 g grated cheese
- Mayonnaise
- Salt

Steps to Cook

1. Boil the corn for 10 minutes.
2. On a griddle add butter and brown the corn.
3. Then paint them with mayonnaise and add the chopped chile and grated cheese.

Nutritional Information:

- Calorie: 51
- Protein: 1g
- Fat: 6g
- Carbohydrates: 1g

Chickpeas With Spinach

Servings: 1

Preparation time: 5 minutes

Cook time: 10-15 minutes

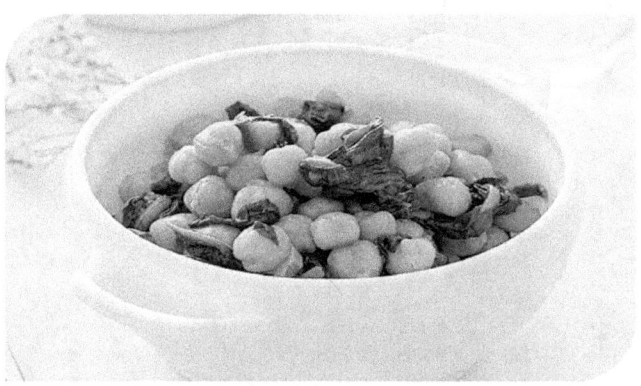

Ingredients

- Extra virgin olive oil
- 10 cloves of garlic
- 2 to 4 tablespoons of sweet paprika
- ½ lbs. spinach
- 1 lbs. cooked chickpeas
- Salt
- White wine

Steps to Cook

1. The day before, cook the chickpeas. Once tender, reserve them in the fridge until the next day.
2. In a low saucepan add a good stream of extra virgin olive oil, cover the bottom and add the chopped garlic until they start to take on a light color.
3. Add the paprika, stir well and add the chopped spinach, a splash of white wine and a pinch of salt. Let cook for 5 minutes.
4. Finally incorporate the chickpeas and stir, let cook for 5 more minutes and serve.

Nutritional Information:

- Calorie: 209
- Protein: 6.8g
- Fat: 8.1g
- Carbohydrates: 28.5g

Rice With Vegetables

Servings: 2-4
Preparation time: 5 minutes
Cook time: 30-40 minutes

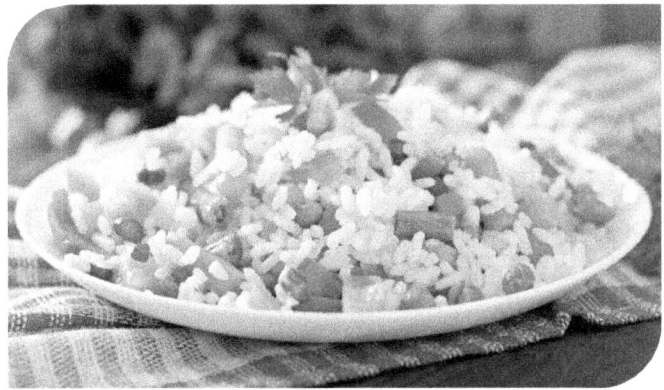

Ingredients

- 1 cup of rice
- 2 cups of water
- Pepper
- Zucchini
- Mushrooms
- Onion
- Green pepper
- Soy sauce
- Crispy Onion

Steps to Cook

1. First cut the vegetables and fry the vegetables until the onion is transparent, without toasting.
2. In the same frying pan add the rice to sauté for a minute, while put the two measures of water to heat in the microwave, to add them to the already hot rice. After a minute or so, add the water little by little with the medium heat. If you see that the water is consumed and the rice is still hard, add a little more, also hot, so that the rice does not end up sticky.
3. When it is almost ready, a splash of soy sauce, turn off the heat and let the rice rest, covering the pan.
4. Once on the plate, you can add a little crispy onion on top.

Nutritional Information:

- Calorie: 219.8
- Protein: 4g
- Fat: 4g
- Carbohydrates: 43g

Integral Rice With Heura

Servings: 2-4
Preparation time: 5 minutes
Cook time: 30-40 minutes

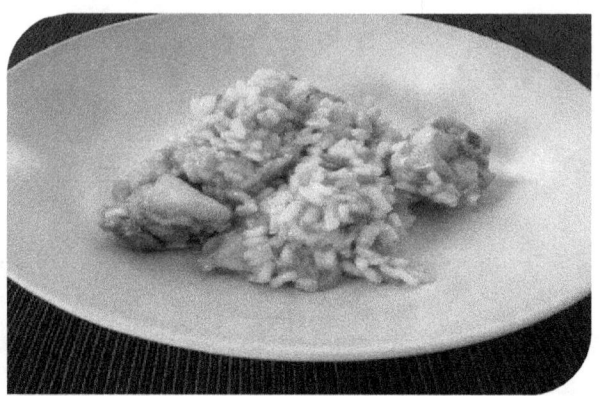

Ingredients

- ½ lbs. of brown rice
- ½ lbs. Heura bites original flavor
- 1 lb. of vegetable ratatouille
- 5 cups of vegetable broth
- 3 oz. canned peas
- 1 pinch of hot paprika
- 1 pinch garlic powder
- 1 pinch of pepper
- 1 pinch of turmeric
- Salt

Steps to Cook

1. Sauté Heura's bites in a large skillet with a little oil and sauté until they start to brown. Add the ratatouille. Let it be done together with the bites for 2 or 3 minutes.
2. Add the brown rice, the peas, and then the vegetable stock. Add the paprika, garlic powder, turmeric and a little herbal salt.
3. Let it cook over medium-low heat until all the broth is absorbed, you do not need to stir it much. If you see that the rice is getting hard, you can add a little more water until it is to your liking.
4. Once ready let it rest for a few minutes and then stir all the rice well to mix the ingredients

Nutritional Information:

- Calorie: 218
- Protein: 4.5g
- Fat: 1.6g
- Carbohydrates: 45.8g

Couscous With Vegetables

Servings: 2-4
Preparation time: 5 minutes
Cook time: 10 minutes

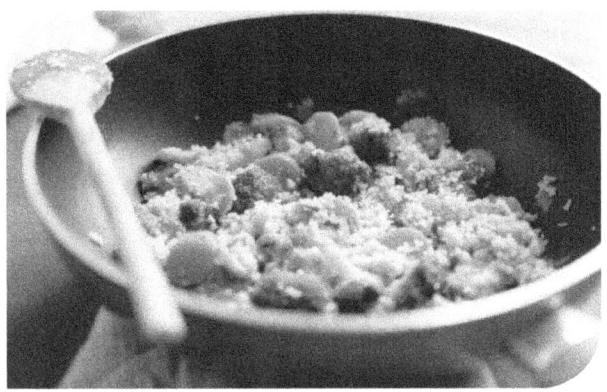

Ingredients

- 1 zucchini
- 2 carrots
- 1 fresh chive
- A handful of cherry tomatoes
- Extra virgin olive oil
- Vegetables soup
- Parsley
- Salt
- ½ lbs. couscous
- ½ lbs. vegetable broth

Steps to Cook

1. Sauté the onion, carrot, zucchini and cherry tomatoes with two tablespoons of extra virgin olive oil and salt. Stir occasionally and cook until vegetables are tender, but not too overdue.
2. Heat the vegetable stock in a saucepan. Before it starts to boil, remove the saucepan from the heat and add the couscous. Let it hydrate for a while (about 10 minutes), add a tablespoon of oil and mix well so that the couscous is loose.
3. The recipe can be eaten both hot and cold, both ways it is delicious.

Nutritional Information:

- Calorie: 249.2
- Protein: 6.4g
- Fat: 7.2g
- Carbohydrates: 40.5g

Sarraceno Wheat With Curry

Servings: 2-4

Preparation time: 15 minutes

Cook time: 30-40 minutes

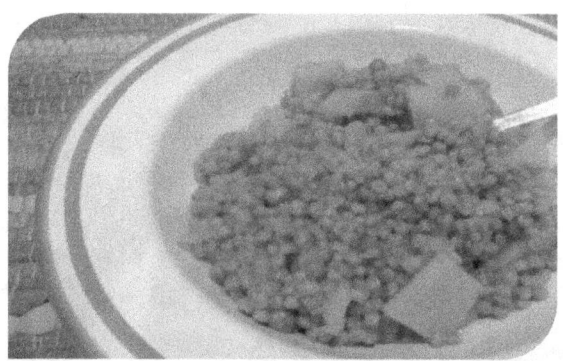

Ingredients

- 1 cup buckwheat
- 2 cups of vegetable broth
- 1 clove garlic
- ½ diced eggplant
- Virgin olive oil
- Salt

For the curry sauce:

- 1 clove garlic
- 1 tbsp virgin olive oil
- 2 glasses of almond milk
- 2 tbsp cornstarch
- 2 tsp of curry powder

Steps to Cook

1. First, prepare the buckwheat. Put the pot with water on the fire when it starts to boil add the wheat and cover. Leave on low heat about 20-25 minutes.
2. Meanwhile, cut the eggplant into cubes and put with a little oil and a clove of garlic in the pan over medium heat until it is soft and golden. If you feel like it, you can use other or various vegetables, onions, zucchini ... or any other that you have in the fridge and you need to take advantage of it.
3. To make the sauce put the oil in a saucepan along with the minced garlic clove, add the cornstarch and mix. Then put the almond milk and the curry and let it reduce over low heat.
4. When you have all the ingredients assemble the plate and enjoy the buckwheat curry!

Nutritional Information:

- Calorie: 140
- Protein: 12g
- Fat: 0.5g
- Carbohydrates: 23g

Chapter 6

Vegetables

Baked Mushrooms

Servings: 1
Preparation time: 5 minutes
Cook time: 5 minutes

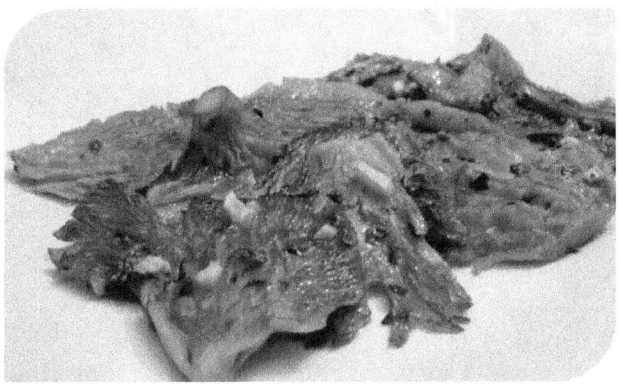

Ingredients

- Mushrooms, quantity to taste
- Olive oil
- Soy sauce
- Salt, garlic, parsley

Steps to Cook

1. Preheat the oven to 180°C more or less and all you have to do is put a little oil in the oven tray.
2. Place the mushrooms in it and then sprinkle over the salt, garlic and parsley and a drizzle of oil on top.
3. Put in the oven until the mushrooms are a little brown and then you can accompany them with a little soy sauce. They are delicious and it doesn't take long.

Nutritional Information:

- Calorie: 164
- Protein: 3.4g
- Fat: 14g
- Carbohydrates: 8.5g

Fried Sweet Potato

Servings: 1
Preparation time: 5 minutes
Cook time: 10-15 minutes

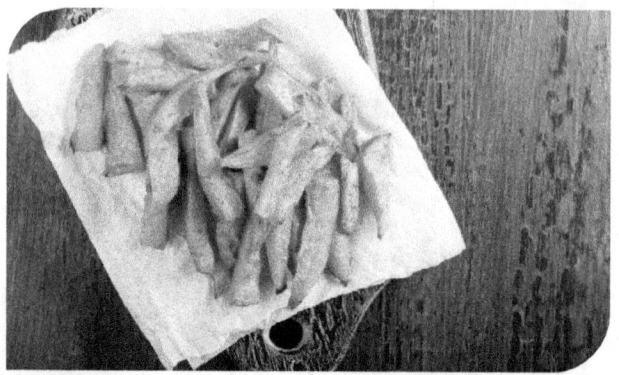

Ingredients

- sweet potato
- frying oil
- Salt

Steps to Cook

1. Wash and peel the sweet potatoes, and cut them into sticks of a similar thickness and length, so that they cook at the same time.
2. Heat plenty of oil in a high-sided saucepan. When the oil is hot, add a little of the sweet potatoes, being careful not to burn yourself; they should be covered with the oil, it is better to make more batches of less sweet potato so that they brown well.
3. Every so often stir with a slotted spoon so that they cook evenly, when they are golden remove with a slotted spoon, drain on absorbent paper, salt and serve very hot.

Nutritional Information:

- Calorie: 173
- Protein: 3g
- Fat: 0.2g
- Carbohydrates: 40g

Fried Cauliflowers

Servings: 2-3
Preparation time: 5 minutes
Cook time: 18 minutes

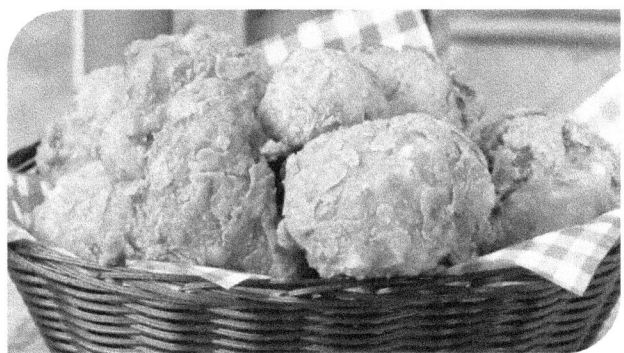

Ingredients

- 1 cauliflower
- 2 cups wheat flour
- 1 tbsp baking powder
- 2 tbsp salt
- 1 tbsp cumin
- ½ tsp pepper
- ½ tsp garlic salt
- ¼ tsp paprika
- Ta tsp spices
- 1 ¾ cup of mineral water
- ¼ cup oil

Steps to Cook

1. Preheat the oven to 360°F.
2. You cut the cauliflower in half and with your hands separate the foils.
3. About the size of a wing, they are placed on a baking sheet.
4. Mix the dry ingredients in a bowl, when well-integrated.
5. Add the liquids and mix until you have a homogeneous consistency.
6. Dip each foil into the mixture and return to the baking sheet.
7. Bake for 18 minutes.
8. When leaving the oven, they can be fried in vegetable oil and when leaving the fryer add sauce of your choice, bbq, buffalo, etc.

Nutritional Information:

- Calorie: 146
- Protein: 3.3g
- Fat: 10g
- Carbohydrates: 10g

Baked Artichoke

Servings: 12
Preparation time: 5 minutes
Cook time: 40 minutes

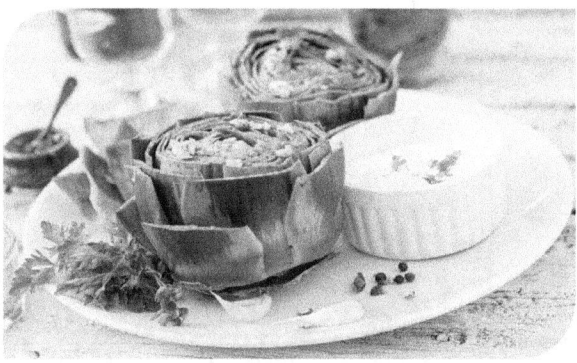

Ingredients

- 12 artichokes
- 1 lemon
- Extra virgin olive oil
- Salt

Steps to Cook

1. Wash the artichokes and with a knife cut the stem and a little of the base, this will make them stand up without problems.
2. Also cut the top tip and with your hand or with the blade of a knife, press a little to open them.
3. Put in a baking tray and on top put a little lemon juice, salt and extra virgin olive oil.
4. Put in the oven, preheated, at 180°C for about 40 minutes.
5. Take out and all that remains is to enjoy these delicious baked Artichokes.

Nutritional Information:

- Calorie: 212.7
- Protein: 5.8g
- Fat: 13.9g
- Carbohydrates: 24.2g

Vegan Pancakes With Vegetables

Servings: 2
Preparation time: 5 minutes
Cook time: 5 minutes

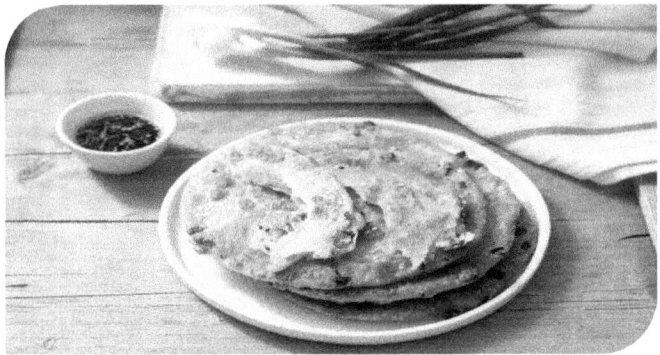

Ingredients

For the pancakes
- ½ cup chickpea flour
- ½ cup of water

For filling:
- 1 large zuchini
- 2 carrots
- 1 onion
- Garlic
- Salt
- Turmeric
- Pepper
- Coconut milk or other vegetable cream

Steps to Cook

1. Place the chickpea flour and water in a deep bowl and beat to integrate well with an electric or wire whisk.
2. Heat over medium-low heat in a medium nonstick skillet to cook pancakes. Add a few drops of oil to prevent the dough from sticking. Once the pan is very hot, add a few tablespoons of the preparation to make the first pancake. Once the edges begin to peel off, turn it over to cook on the other side. Repeat the process two more times. Reserve the pancakes.

For the filling:

3. Chop the onion and cook it in a pan with oil until it becomes transparent. Meanwhile, peel and cut the carrot and zuchini into cubes of the desired size. Also chop the garlic. Pour the garlic, carrot and zuchini into the pan and cook for a few minutes until the vegetables are tender. Finally add turmeric, pepper and serve.

Nutritional Information:

- Calorie: 198.2
- Protein: 8.6g
- Fat: 6.2g
- Carbohydrates: 30.4g

Chocolate Oatmeal

Servings: 2
Preparation time: 5 minutes
Cook time: 5 minutes

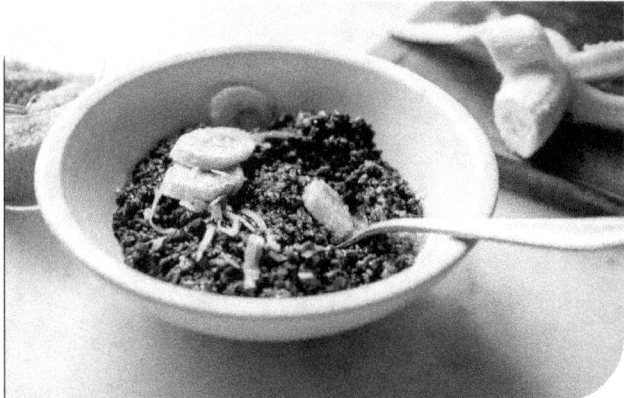

Ingredients

- 2 cups divided unsweetened plant-based milk
- 5-6 seedless dates
- ¾ cup oat flakes
- 1 ½ tablespoon cocoa powder
- ½ teaspoon cinnamon
- 1 tablespoon chia seeds
- Fresh or thawed strawberries or cherries

Steps to Cook

1. Combine one cup of the almond milk with the dates in a blender until the dried fruits are crushed well and the consistency is creamy.
2. Transfer the mixture along with the additional cup of milk to a medium saucepan and add the rest of the ingredients except the fruits.
3. Bring to a simmer and cook over medium heat until thickened, about 15 minutes.
4. Add additional milk if the oatmeal is too thick for your taste.
5. Serve with bananas.

Nutritional Information:

- Calorie: 369.1
- Protein: 8.4g
- Fat: 4.5g
- Carbohydrates: 70.5g

Vegetarian Tacos

Servings: 4
Preparation time: 5 minutes
Cook time: 5 minutes

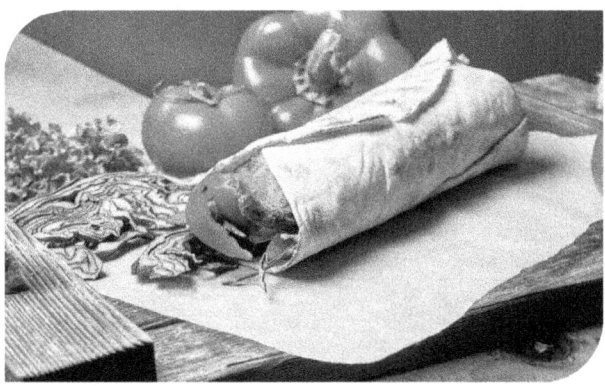

Ingredients

- 1 tbsp of vegetable oil
- ½ cup red onion
- ½ cups green or red bell pepper
- 15.25 oz black beans unsalted
- 15.25 oz. corn kernels, unsalted
- 1 teaspoon of ground cumin
- 2 cups of water
- 1 package Taco Rice
- 2 tablespoons fresh coriander

Steps to Cook

4. Heat oil in large nonstick skillet over medium-high heat and cook onion, bell pepper, beans, corn, and cumin, stirring occasionally, for about 5 minutes. Stir and reserve.
5. Add the water and Taco Rice in the same pan and bring to a boil. Reduce heat to low and simmer, covered, for 7 minutes or until rice is tender.
6. Incorporate the vegetables; Let stand covered for 2 minutes. Add the coriander. If desired, serve with your favorite taco side dishes, such as diced avocado, tomato, onion, grated cheese, lime wedges, sour cream, sliced radishes, and hot sauce; now they are delicious. Enjoy it!

Nutritional Information:

- Calorie: 280
- Protein: 12g
- Fat: 10g
- Carbohydrates: 37g

Mushroom Leek Quiche

Servings: 8
Preparation time: 20 minutes
Cook time: 20 minutes

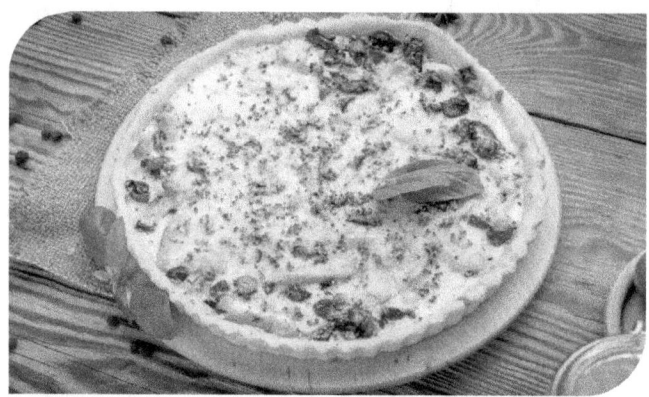

Ingredients

For the mass:
- ½ lbs. whole wheat flour
- 4 tablespoons of oil
- ½ cup of water
- 1 pinch of salt

For the filling:
- 2 leeks
- 2 cups of mushrooms
- 2 small onion
- 1 clove garlic
- 6 cherry tomatoes
- Salt, pepper and spices to taste
- 6 tbsp of chickpea flour
- 18 tablespoons of water
- 1 teaspoon of vinegar

Steps to Cook

For the mass:
1. In a bowl place the flour, oil, water and salt and mix well to form smooth dough.
2. Roll it out on a previously oiled cake pan or upholstered with vegetable paper. Pinch the dough with a fork.
3. Bake at 360°F for 10 minutes until slightly cooked.

For the filling:
4. In a frying pan, sauté the onions, leeks and garlic in olive oil. Add the mushrooms, salt, pepper and spices and sauté for a few more minutes.
5. Once it is well cooked, pour into a bowl and let it cool down a bit.
6. In another bowl place the chickpea flour, vinegar and water and form an egg-like cream.
7. Add this mixture to the vegetables and mix well.
8. Pour it over the previously cooked dough, decorate with cherrys cut in half and take to the oven for 10-15 more minutes until the edges of the dough are well cooked and the mixture of chickpea flour, vinegar and water has linked the ingredients.

Nutritional Information:

- Calorie: 245
- Protein: 6.8g
- Fat: 16.4g
- Carbohydrates: 18.3g

Vegan Cheese Fingers

Servings: 2-4
Preparation time: 5 minutes
Cook time: 15-20 minutes

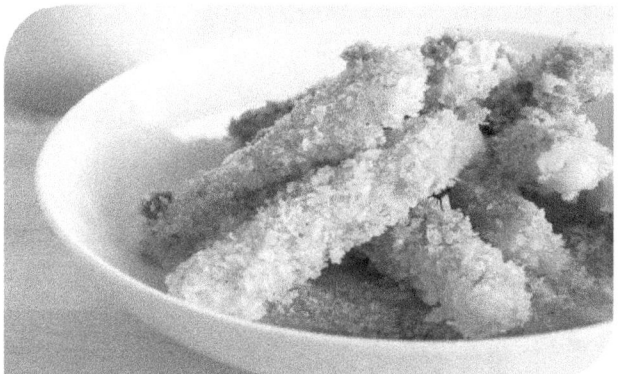

Ingredients

- 1 pack of ½ lbs. vegan Mozzarella
- ½ cup tempura flour
- 1 cup panko
- Garlic powder
- Black pepper powder
- Parsley
- Salt

Steps to Cook

1. First cook the lentils. Put about 1 cup and a pinch of salt. Cook about 15-20 minutes over low heat.
2. Drain them and let them warm a little. Meanwhile, you can squeeze the juice of half a lemon.
3. Put the lentils in the mixer glass, add the tahini, the lemon juice, the oil and the spices and beat until you have the texture that you like the most.
4. Keep in mind that depending on the power you choose in your mixer it will have more or less consistency. So, to taste. Test if it is well of salt and that's it! You can present with a splash of olive oil and a little paprika from Vera.

Nutritional Information:

- Calorie: 45
- Protein: 1g
- Fat: 0.4g
- Carbohydrates: 9g

Escalivada

Servings: 2-4
Preparation time: 5 minutes
Cook time: 50 minutes

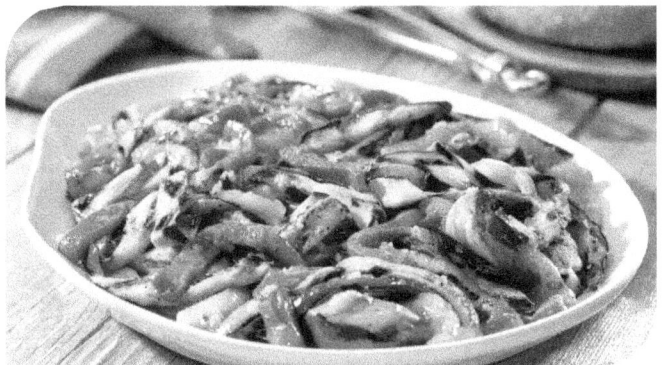

Ingredients

- 2 aubergines
- 3 onions
- 4 or 5 tomatoes
- 2 red bell peppers
- 1 head of garlic
- Salt
- Extra virgin olive oil
- 2 or 3 cloves of garlic

Steps to Cook

1. Wash everything under running water and place on a cookie sheet. Prick the eggplants with a knife so they do not burst. Add a little extra virgin olive oil and salt on top, although there are those who do not put anything. Once the oven is preheated to 180°C, put the tray in and leave to bake for about 50 minutes. Halfway through cooking we will turn them over so that they cook evenly.
2. When the vegetables are cooked, remove the tray from the oven and immediately peel and cut into strips. To extract the garlic, you just have to press the skin and they will come out completely, add all the juice that is in the tray. Once cold, season with extra virgin olive oil, salt and finely chopped garlic.

Nutritional Information:

- Calorie: 80
- Protein: 1g
- Fat: 6g
- Carbohydrates: 5g

Green Beans With Tomato And Textured Soybean

Servings: 2
Preparation time: 5 minutes
Cook time: 35 minutes

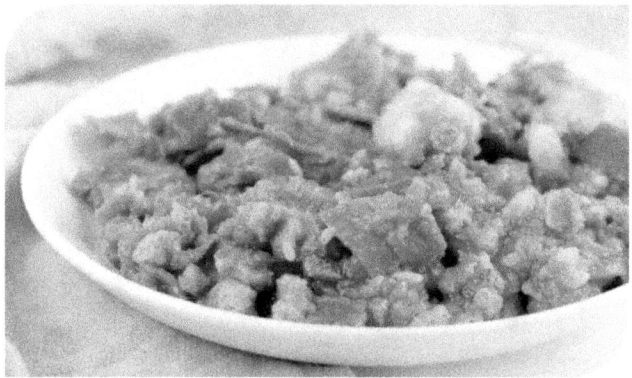

Ingredients

- 1 lbs. green beans
- 1 potato
- 1 glass of textured soybean
- 1 lbs. tomato crushed
- Onion powder
- Extra virgin olive oil
- Get out

Steps to Cook

1. Bring water to a boil and put the diced potatoes. Meanwhile, wash and prepare the beans by removing the sides with a peeler, cutting the spikes off the ends and then dicing.
2. Soak the textured soy in hot water for about 10 minutes. Going back to the potatoes, when the water starts to boil add the beans and let it cook for about 20 minutes.
3. Once the soy is soft, drain it and sauté it with olive oil and a little onion powder.
4. Then, remove the pot from the heat and drain the beans and potato and add them to the pan with the soy. Put the crushed tomato and stir. Let it all go together for about 5 minutes and you're done!
5. If you serve a plate of olive oil on top of the dish, it is delicious.

Nutritional Information:

- Calorie: 135.1
- Protein: 4g
- Fat: 3.5g
- Carbohydrates: 22.1g

Vegetable Tempura

Servings: 2-4
Preparation time: 15 minutes
Cook time: 5-10 minutes

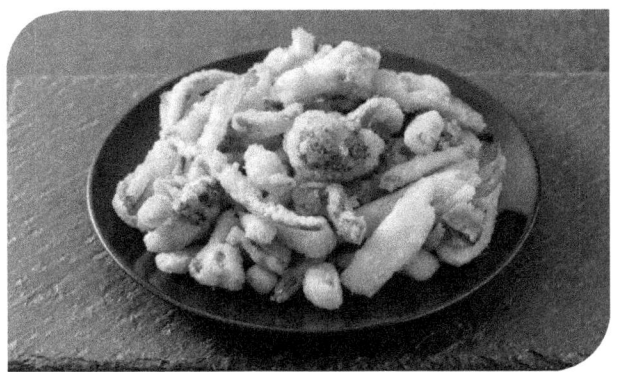

Ingredients

- Tempura flour
- Very cold water
- Soy sauce
- Zucchini
- Eggplant
- Onion
- Carrot
- Oil

Steps to Cook

1. Tempura is very easy to prepare, you have to have very cold water and simply add 2/3 of tempura flour to each part of water. Use a glass as a reference: a glass of cold water + 2/3 of the same glass of flour. Mix it well with a fork and voila.
2. Wash and cut the vegetables: the eggplant and the zucchini in very thin slices, the onion in slices, but a little thicker so that they do not break when removing the rings and the carrot type "sticks".
3. While preparing the tempura, put the oil to heat and the only thing to do afterwards is to sink the vegetables in the tempura and in the pan until they are golden brown. With a medium-high heat, the carrot is not too hard. Put on a plate with kitchen paper, so that it absorbs the excess oil and then on the tray, you accompany it with soy sauce.

Nutritional Information:

- Calorie: 53
- Protein: 0.8g
- Fat: 3.8g
- Carbohydrates: 4.2g

Seitan With Peas Sauce

Servings: 2-4
Preparation time: 15 minutes
Cook time: 15-20 minutes

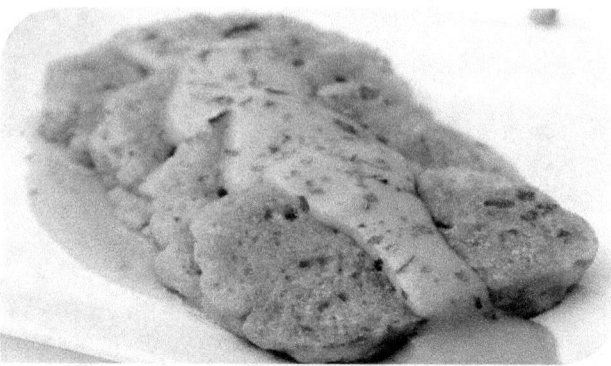

Ingredients

- 1 glass of wheat gluten
- 1 glass with half water and half soy sauce
- 1 tsp of garlic powder
- 1 teaspoon salt
- 1 strip of kombu seaweed

For the sauce:

- ½ lbs. of frozen peas
- ¾ cup of vegetable broth
- 1 teaspoon of flour
- Salt and pepper to taste
- Chopped parsley

Steps to Cook

For the seitan:

1. Put the wheat gluten in a large bowl, add 1 tsp of garlic powder and a pinch of salt and stir. On the other hand, in the same glass with which you have measured the gluten put half of water and half of soy and mix.
2. Then, gradually pour the water over the wheat gluten and knead until everything is compacted. You will see that a very flexible and non-sticky mass almost forms, almost like chewing gum. Shapes into a ball.
3. Reserve and put a pot with enough water to cover the seitan ball and add a strip of kombu seaweed. When it boils, add the seitan and let it cook for about 45 minutes. Remove from the heat, drain the seitan and let it warm. If you see that it is not well done inside when cutting it, nothing happens to put it back a few more minutes in the pot once filleted.
4. For the sauce, simply defrost the peas and beat with the broth. Then strain so that there is a fine sauce without skins. Put in a saucepan with a little salt and pepper to taste and add a teaspoon of flour so that the sauce thickens a little (optional). Let it boil for a couple of minutes and remove. While you can brown the seitan a little.

5. Now all that remains is to plaster the seitan with a pea sauce and sprinkle a little chopped parsley. And to enjoy!

Nutritional Information:

- Calorie: 141
- Protein: 20g
- Fat: 2g
- Carbohydrates: 10g

Tofu And Cereal Wraps

Servings: 2-4
Preparation time: 5 minutes
Cook time: 5-10 minutes

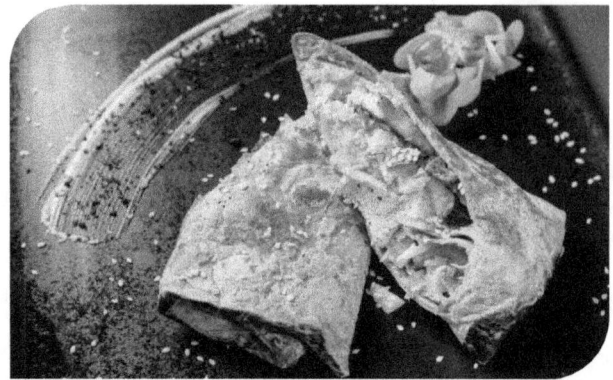

Ingredients

- 2 wheat wraps
- ½ lbs. Tofu
- ½ avocado
- 1 handful of spinach
- 1 ½ oz. spelled
- 1 ½ oz. of assorted seeds
- 2 tablespoons of tomato sauce
- Peppers
- Salt
- Olive oil

Steps to Cook

1. Dice the tofu. Marinate it with a little salt and paprika from the side and sauté over low heat for about 10 minutes, until it is golden and crispy on the outside and soft on the inside.
2. While you are cutting the avocado and washing the spinach. Then heat the wrap in the pan until lightly browned.
3. Spread a tablespoon of tomato in the wrap, add the spinach, tofu, diced avocado and several tablespoons of spelled and seeds.
4. Close and go! Cut and closed them with a wooden skewer to make it easier to eat them.

Nutritional Information:

- Calorie: 360
- Protein: 40g
- Fat: 6g
- Carbohydrates: 15g

Asturian Vegan Tortos

Servings: 4-6
Preparation time: 5 minutes
Cook time: 5-10 minutes

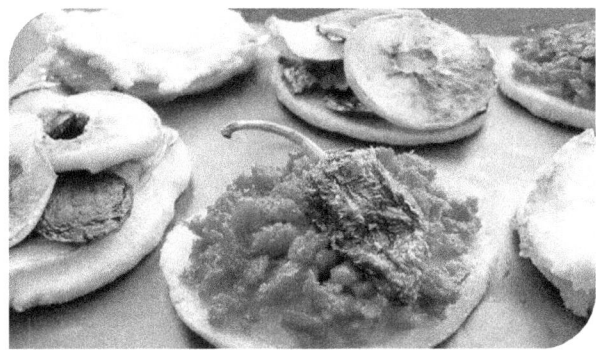

Ingredients

For the mass:
- ½ liter of water
- ½ kilo of cornmeal
- 1 pinch of salt

For the filling:
- Textured soybeans
- Onion
- Zucchini
- Ketchup
- Mushrooms
- Pepper
- Paprika
- Salt and oil

Steps to Cook

1. Heat the water, without boiling, and then add a pinch of salt. Put the corn flour in a large bowl and add the water little by little while kneading with your hands. The texture that remains is very moldable. Make small balls and crush them on a cloth rag. Fry them with very hot oil until they are golden.
2. **For soybean**: Hydrate soybean in water for a quarter of an hour or so. Fry the onion, pepper, zucchini with a little salt. After draining the soybeans, add it and let it be done with the rest of the ingredients and almost at the end add a little tomato sauce and a little bell pepper.
3. **For those with mushrooms**: Clean the mushrooms and cut them, the same with the zucchini and fry with a little salt.

Nutritional Information:

- Calorie: 280
- Protein: 12g
- Fat: 10g
- Carbohydrates: 37g

Rustic Potatoes With Turmeric

Servings: 4
Preparation time: 5 minutes
Cook time: 40 minutes

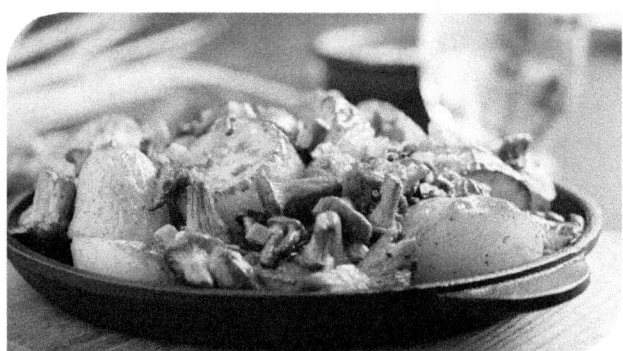

Ingredients

- 3 large potatoes
- 1 tsp turmeric
- 2 tablespoons nutritional yeast
- 1 tsp pink salt
- Pepper
- Olive oil

Steps to Cook

1. Cut the potatoes into wedges and pour them into a bowl. Season with turmeric, yeast, oil (1/4 cup) and pepper. Mix well with your hands and place them on a plate.
2. Cook in the oven.
3. When they are golden, add the salt.
4. This allows them to stay even crispier done!
5. Put in some fresh parsley.

Nutritional Information:

- Calorie: 110
- Protein: 2g
- Fat: 6g
- Carbohydrates: 13g

Sweet And Sour Tofu With Peppers

Servings: 4
Preparation time: 5 minutes
Cook time: 5-10 minutes

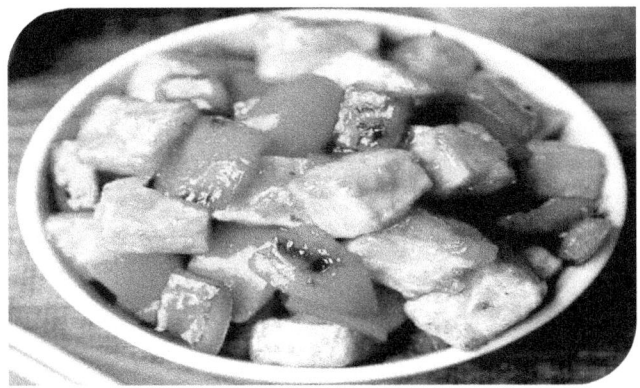

Ingredients

- 1 lbs. firm tofu
- 1 red pepper
- 1 yellow bell pepper cut into bite-size pieces
- 3 tbsp of virgin olive oil
- fine corn flour to coat

For the sweet and sour sauce:

- 2 tbsp of honey
- 1 tbsp of ketchup
- 1 tbsp soy sauce
- 3 tbsp of vinegar
- 1 pinch of salt
- 0 ml of water

Steps to Cook

1. In a bowl we beat all the ingredients of the sauce, until they are well mixed. You will already have the tofu strained and cut into cubes.
2. Pass it through the fine cornmeal and sauté in a pan with the olive oil, until all the sides are golden brown. Withdraw and reserve.
3. In the same oil, sauté the peppers for a few minutes, they should still be crisp.
4. Put the tofu back in the pan, pour the sauce on top and stir over the heat until the sauce is well distributed. Remove from heat and serve.

Nutritional Information:

- Calorie: 207.2
- Protein: 18.1g
- Fat: 11.7g
- Carbohydrates: 12.7g

Spicy Tofu With Honey And Sesame

Servings: 2-4
Preparation time: 10 minutes
Cook time: 3-5 minutes

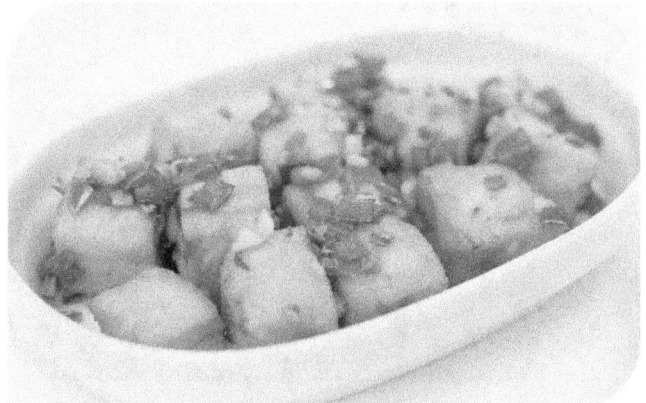

Ingredients

- 1 lbs. cubed regular or firm tofu
- 1 clove garlic, minced
- 2 tbsp of Mexican hot sauce
- 1 tbsp soy sauce
- 2 tbsp of honey
- 1 tbsp of apple cider vinegar
- 3 tbsp of extra virgin olive oil
- fine corn flour to coat
- 1 tbsp of sesame seeds

Steps to Cook

1. In a bowl, beat the hot sauce, soy sauce, honey, garlic and vinegar until well mixed. You will already have the tofu strained and cut into cubes.
2. Pass it through the fine corn flour and sauté in a frying pan with the olive oil, until all the sides are golden brown.
3. Add the sauce and cook 3 more minutes. Remove from heat, sprinkle with sesame seeds and serve.

Nutritional Information:

- Calorie: 576
- Protein: 20.1g
- Fat: 46.3g
- Carbohydrates: 27.5g

Bimi Toast With Beet Hummus

Servings: 4
Preparation time: 15 minutes
Cook time: 5-10 minutes

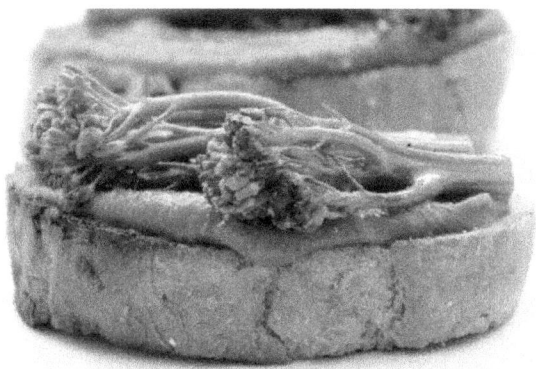

Ingredients

- Bimi
- Rye bread
- ½ lbs. cooked chickpeas
- Cumin grain
- ½ lemon
- ½ lbs. cooked beets
- Extra virgin olive oil

Steps to Cook

1. Prepare the hummus like any other traditional version. Put the drained chickpeas in the mixer and then add the beets and beat until it is uniform. Add the juice of half a lemon, a splash of oil, salt, garlic powder and a splash of olive oil.
2. Once you have the beet hummus to your liking, prepare the bimi. Bimi is a vegetable halfway between broccoli and a type of oriental cabbage. It is very easy to cook, if you put it in the pan, in 3 or 4 minutes it will be ready.
3. To assemble the toasts, toast the bread on one side and once it was ready, add the hummus and then place on top the Bimi that you had previously sautéed and ready!

Nutritional Information:

- Calorie: 50.1
- Protein: 2g
- Fat: 2.5g
- Carbohydrates: 5g

Vegan Barbecue Pizza

Servings: 4
Preparation time: 30 minutes
Cook time: 30-40 minutes

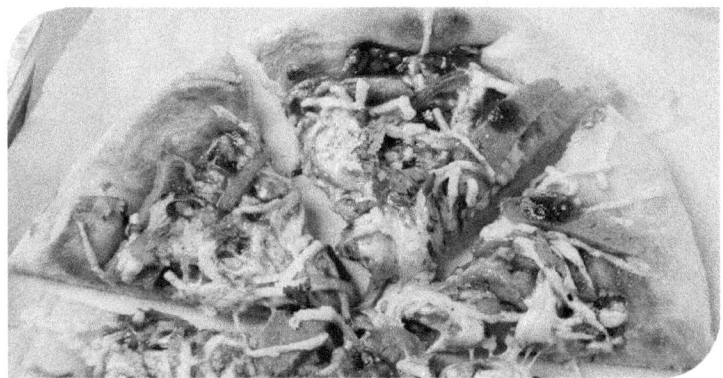

Ingredients

For the base:
- ½ lbs. of pizza flour
- ½ cup warm water
- 3 oil tablespoons
- 1 pinch of salt
- 1 pinch of sugar

For the Barbecue:
- 1 ½ oz. of textured soybeans
- ½ onion
- ¼ green pepper
- ¼ red pepper
- 1 cup crushed tomato
- ½ cup of vegan barbecue sauce
- Vegan cheese
- Oregano and salt

Steps to Cook

1. **For the dough**: Mix the flour with the salt and sugar and then add the water and oil. Knead until smooth, flexible dough remains. Let stand for at least half an hour in a covered bowl. I always put a cup of boiled water under the bowl to keep it warm.
2. **For the barbec**ue: Soak the soy for at least 10 minutes. While cutting the onion and pepper. Put a little olive oil in the pan and fry the vegetables for about 5 minutes. When they start to soften add the well-drained textured soybeans, sauté and then add the tomato. Stir well and finally put the barbecue sauce and let it cook over very low heat.
3. Roll out the dough, which will have grown enough, and give it the shape to bake. With a spoon, put the barbecue over the base of the pizza leaving a not very thick layer. Finally put in the oven preheated to 200°C and leave until the edges begin to brown.

Nutritional Information:

- Calorie: 259
- Protein: 7g
- Fat: 1g
- Carbohydrates: 55g

Chickpea Pilaf

Servings: 4

Preparation time: 5 minutes

Cook time: 30-35 minutes

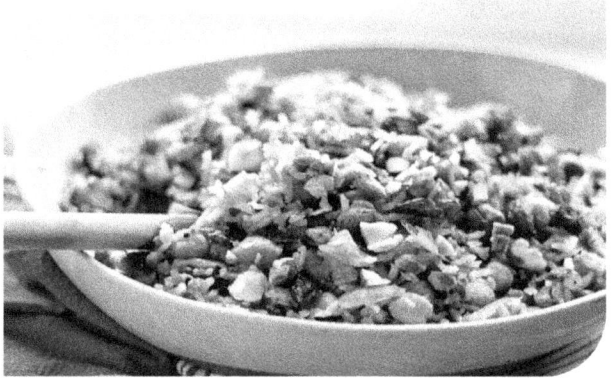

Ingredients

- 1 ½ cups tomatoes
- 1/3 cup of a chopped red onion
- ¼ cup chopped parsley
- ¼ cup chopped fresh mint leaves
- 1 tbsp of olive oil
- 15.5 oz. chickpeas, rinsed and drained
- 1 garlic clove, minced
- 1 package of Rice Pilaf
- 3 tbsp crumbled feta cheese

Steps to Cook

1. Mix the tomatoes, onion, parsley, and mint in a small bowl. If you wish, you can season with salt. Reservation.
2. Heat the olive oil in a large nonstick skillet over medium-high heat. If desired, season the chickpeas with salt and pepper and cook, stirring frequently, until golden brown, about 4 minutes. Add the garlic and cook until it begins to release an aroma, for about 30 seconds. Remove the chickpeas and reserve.
3. Prepare the Rice Pilaf in the same pan, following the instructions on the package. Add the tomato and chickpea mixture and cover with the feta cheese.

Nutritional Information:

- Calorie: 364.5
- Protein: 11g
- Fat: 7.3g
- Carbohydrates: 65g

Vegan Potato and Cauliflower Quiche

Servings: 4

Preparation time: 10 minutes

Cook time: 30-40 minutes

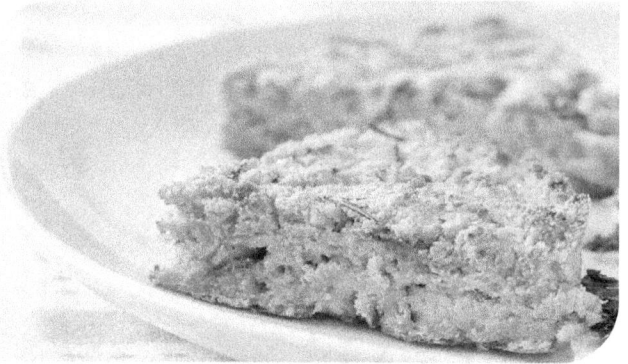

Ingredients

- 1 sheet of shortcrust pastry
- 1 broccoli
- 1 cauliflower
- 1 onion
- 2 tablespoons of flour
- 1 slice of vegan mozzarella cheese
- 1 dash of vegetable broth
- Extra virgin olive oil
- Salt

Steps to Cook

1. Boil the broccoli and cauliflower, cut into small pieces, for about 3 to 4 minutes. While poaching the chopped onion in olive oil and adding a pinch of salt, let it soften for 5-7 minutes over low heat.
2. Then add the broccoli and cauliflower to the pan where you have the onion and mash a little with the spatula itself. Mix well so that the flavors melt well and correct salt. Add the two tablespoons of flour and stir. Add a squirt of vegetable broth.
3. Remove from the heat and pour over the dough that you have previously placed in a mold or greased with a little oil.
4. Arrange your filling evenly throughout the quiche dough, add a little vegan cheese and bake at 360°F for 30-40 minutes. When the edges start to turn golden it will be ready.

Nutritional Information:

- Calorie: 213.7
- Protein: 11.5g
- Fat: 14.8g
- Carbohydrates: 10.5g

Vegan Meatballs Of Brown Rice

Servings: 2-4

Preparation time: 5 minutes

Cook time: 15 minutes

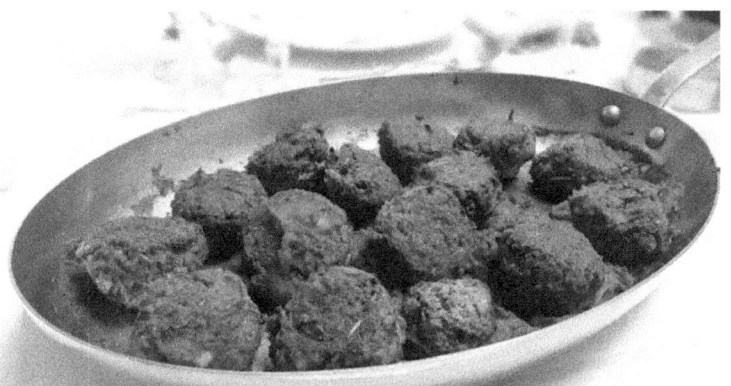

Ingredients

- 1 cup cooked brown
- 1 large onion
- 1 clove garlic
- 1 large carrot
- ½ cup pumpkin
- 1 handful of parsley
- ½ cup oatmeal
- Salt and pepper to taste

Steps to Cook

1. Sauté the onion with the garlic and the fine grated carrot. Reserve.
2. Cook the pumpkin in the oven with soy sauce and oil. Reserve.
3. Put the cooked rice, onion, garlic, carrot, squash and parsley in a food processor.
4. Process to integrate well. Taste and adjust the amount of seasoning.
5. Pour the mixture into a bowl and add the oats. Mix with your hands to form malleable dough to form balls.
6. Arrange on an oiled baking sheet and cook over moderate heat for about 15 minutes, turn them over and continue cooking until golden.

Nutritional Information:

- Calorie: 204.1
- Protein: 8.9g
- Fat: 8.4g
- Carbohydrates: 25.6g

Kentucky Fried Cauliflower

Servings: 2-4

Preparation time: 15 minutes

Cook time: 15-20 minutes

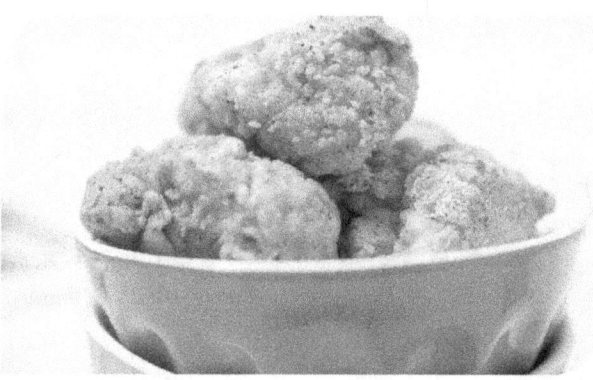

Ingredients

- 2 cups soy milk
- 2 tbsp apple cider vinegar
- 1 cauliflower
- 1 liter of oil for frying
- 2 cups plain flour
- 3 tbsp of salt
- 2 tbsp garlic powder
- 2 tbsp onion powder
- 3 tbsp dry mixed herbs
- 1 tbsp paprika
- 1 tbsp white pepper
- 3 tsp baking soda

Steps to Cook

1. In a small bowl, mix the soy milk and apple cider vinegar. Set aside.
2. Cut the cauliflower into pieces and set aside.
3. Add the oil to a saucepan or deep fryer and bring to medium-high heat.
4. In another small bowl, mix together the flour, salt, garlic powder, onion powder, dried herbs, paprika, pepper, and baking soda.
5. Coat each piece of cauliflower in the soy milk mixture before completely covering the flour mixture, gently removing the excess before carefully adding to the oil.
6. Cook until golden and deep and drain on a paper towel before adding extra salt and serving with your favorite sauce.

Nutritional Information:

- Calorie: 146
- Protein: 3.3g
- Fat: 10g
- Carbohydrates: 10g

Flourless Spinach Pancakes

Servings: 2-4

Preparation time: 5 minutes

Cook time: 10-12 minutes

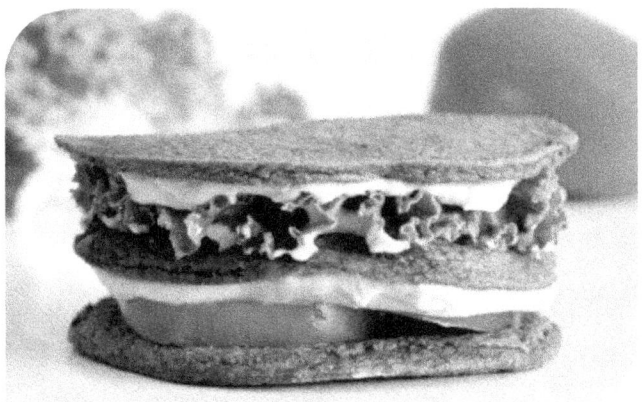

Ingredients

- 1 large bowl of raw spinach
- 2 eggs
- 1 tablespoon of oil
- Salt, pepper and spices to taste

Steps to Cook

1. To prepare spinach pancakes, place the eggs in a bowl, add the salt and spices and beat with the help of a wire whisk or fork.
2. Pour the eggs into the glass of the mixer or food processor along with the raw spinach.
3. Process all ingredients well.
4. Light the stove and place the pan on the fire. Add a tablespoon of oil and wait a few minutes until it is very hot.
5. Pour a quarter of the preparation on the hot skillet and cook for a few minutes on one side. Peel off the edges with the help of a wooden spatula and once it is well cooked on one side, turn it over and leave a few more minutes on the other side. Be careful that it does not burn!
6. Place the crepe on a plate and repeat the previous steps with the rest of the preparation until you make 4 or 5 crepes. The amount will also depend on the thickness desired for each pancake.
7. Fill with steamed vegetables and green salad. Accompany with beet or avocado dressing

Nutritional Information:

- Calorie: 175
- Protein: 10g
- Fat: 5g
- Carbohydrates: 24g

Vegan Ricotta

Servings: 2-4

Preparation time: 5 minutes

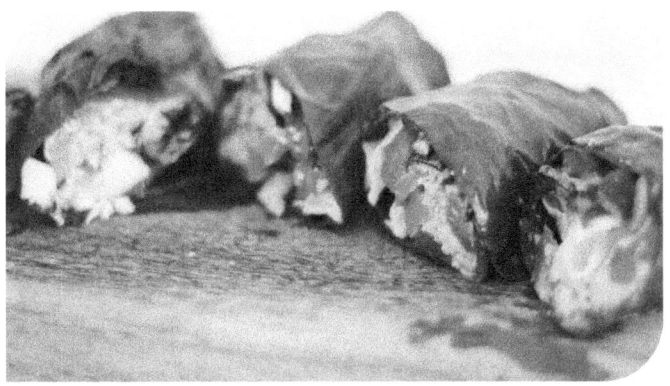

Ingredients

For ricotta

- 1 cup bagasse
- Coconut or olive oil
- 1 tbsp apple or lemon vinegar

For the rolls

- Whole chard leaves
- Red peppers
- Roasted aubergine
- Roasted pumpkin
- White cabbage

Steps to Cook

1. Process the bagasse until it is well crushed. Add 1 tbsp of oil and vinegar or lemon. Salt.
2. Add water little by little until it reaches the consistency of ricotta.
3. Spread the chard leaves.
4. Add ingredients linearly. Roll up.

Nutritional Information:

- Calorie: 317.5
- Protein: 30.7g
- Fat: 5g
- Carbohydrates: 12.3g

Aubergine Sandwich With Hummus

Servings: 2

Preparation time: 5 minutes

Cooking time: 5 minutes

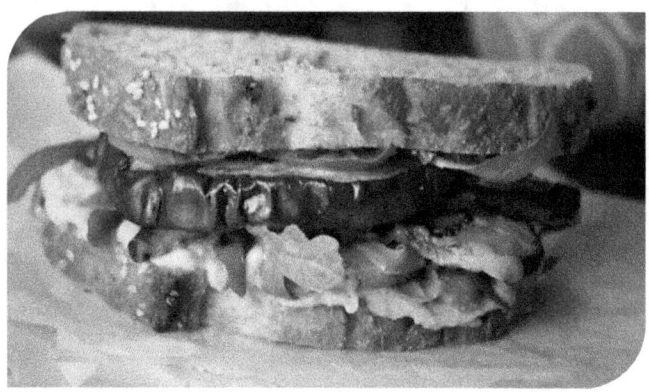

Ingredients

- ½ can of chickpeas drained
- The juice of 2 lemons
- 1 Wholemeal bread
- ¼ cup olive oil and 3 extra tablespoons
- 1 small clove of garlic
- 1 tbsp of tagine
- 1 cup spinach leaves
- 1 tomato in quarters
- ½ sliced eggplant

Steps to Cook

1. Blend the chickpeas with the lemon juice, a cup of olive oil, the garlic and the tagine until obtaining a smooth consistency; season.
2. Season the aubergine and tomato with salt and pepper and grill on a hot griddle with the remaining oil.
3. Toast the bread a little in the oven, spread the hummus and arrange the roasted vegetables on it; finish with the spinach and serve.

Nutritional Information:

- Calorie: 511
- Protein: 13.5g
- Fat: 22.6g
- Carbohydrates: 68.3g

Vegan French Toast

Servings: 2

Preparation time: 5 minutes

Cooking time: 20-25 minutes

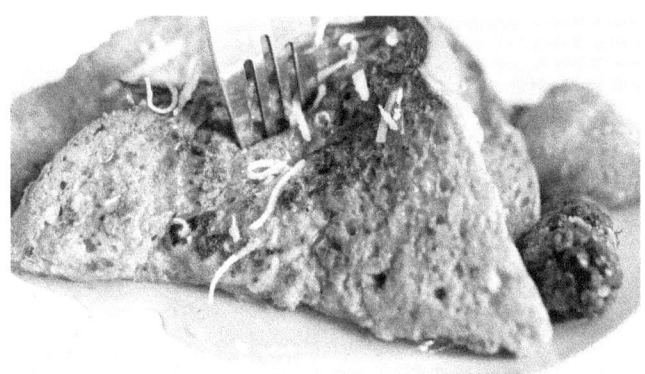

Ingredients

- 4 slices of vegan sliced bread
- ¾ cup coconut milk
- 1 ½ tbsp of muscovado sugar
- ¾ tbsp ground cinnamon
- 1 pinch of sea salt
- 1 teaspoon of vanilla extract
- ¼ cup + 1 tbsp cornstarch

To cook:

- Coconut oil

Steps to Cook

1. In a large bowl mix the coconut milk, sugar, cinnamon, salt, cornstarch and vanilla. Mix until smooth.
2. Heat a frying pan over medium heat, oil well with the oil of your choice.
3. Soak one slice at a time in the liquid mixture you prepared earlier, cover both sides.
4. When the pan is hot, place one of the slices of bread and cook for 2-3 minutes until one side is browned. When it is golden, turn and brown the other side. Repeat this operation with all the slices.
5. Remember to oil the pan between slices to prevent the toasts from sticking.
6. Serve with maple syrup, agave, or chocolate. Accompany with coconut zest and red berries.

Nutritional Information:

- Calorie: 162.2
- Protein: 6.2g
- Fat: 3.4g
- Carbohydrates: 28.2g

Carrot Pancake

Servings: 4

Preparation time: 10 minutes

Cooking time: 2 minutes

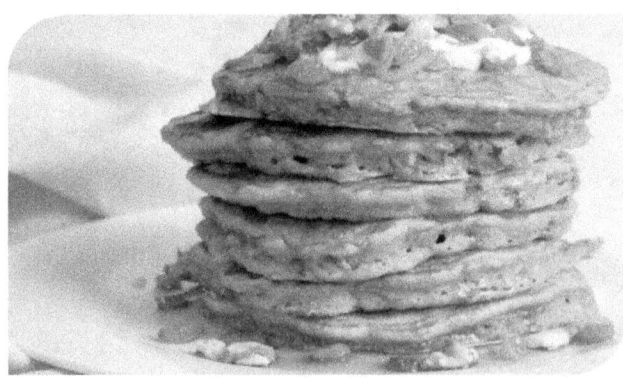

Ingredients

- ½ lbs. whole wheat flour
- 1 tsp of baking powder
- ½ tsp food grade baking soda
- 1 tsp cinnamon powder
- 2 tbsp of cornstarch
- ½ tsp of sea salt
- 1 tsp ground flaxseed
- 1 tsp of apple cider
- ½ tbsp vanilla extract
- ¼ of Cup of agave syrup
- 1 cup coconut milk
- 1 cup of grated carrot

Steps to Cook

1. Mix all the dry ingredients in a large bowl.
2. Add the liquid ingredients, mix well and finally add the grated carrot. Mix until a homogeneous consistency is obtained.
3. Cook in a nonstick skillet over low heat. Put a little oil with the help of a cloth or napkin if you need to prevent the hotcakes from sticking to the surface.
4. Cook each hotcake by pouring the mixture onto the surface of the already hot pan, wait for bubbles to come out on almost the entire surface and turn. Cook for 2 more minutes and repeat the operation until all the mixture is finished.

Nutritional Information:

- Calorie: 323.1
- Protein: 8.6g
- Fat: 7.7g
- Carbohydrates: 55.6g

Revolted Tofu

Servings: 2

Preparation time: 5 minutes

Cooking time: 15 minutes

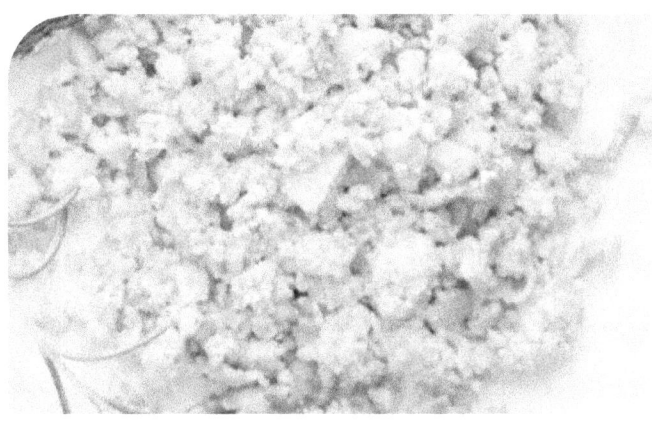

Ingredients

- 1 lb. of extra firm tofu previously drained
- 1 tbsp nutritional yeast
- ½ tbsp garlic powder
- 1 tsp of turmeric powder
- ¼ tsp of sea salt

Steps to Cook

1. Put the tofu in a bowl and with the help of a fork, grind it until you get a texture similar to scrambled eggs. It does not have to be perfect since in the pan you can crush it more if you like.
2. Add the other ingredients and stir well.
3. Put a pan on high heat and wait until it is hot. You can oil the surface a little with the help of a napkin and a few drops of olive oil.
4. Place the tofu in the pan and cook for 5 minutes without stirring. Stir and let cook another 5 minutes. Repeat the operation once more.
5. Serve accompanied by toasted bread.

Nutritional Information:

- Calorie: 177
- Protein: 15.57g
- Fat: 12.19g
- Carbohydrates: 5.36g

Vegetarian Huarache

Servings: 2
Preparation time: 5 minutes
Cooking time: 5 minutes

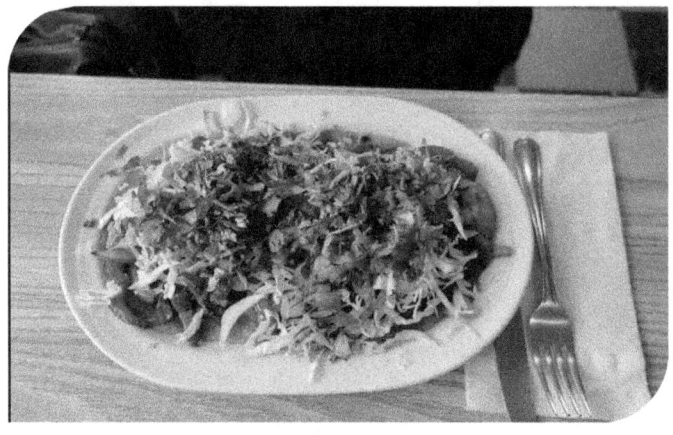

Ingredients

- 2 tbsp of olive oil
- 1 cup yellow bell pepper strips
- 1 cup green pepper strips
- ½ cup sliced onion
- 1 medium bowl of red sauce
- 1 medium bowl of green sauce
- 4 huaraches
- 2 cups of refried beans
- 1 cup lettuce

Steps to Cook

1. In a frying pan, heat the oil and sauté the peppers together with the onion.
2. Heat the sauces separately until they boil. Hold the fire for five minutes, turn it off and set them aside.
3. Heat the huaraches. Spread the beans on them, spoon green and red sauce on top (in each half) and place a little of the pepper mixture on top.
4. Complete with a little lettuce. Serve immediately.

Nutritional Information:

- Calorie: 976
- Protein: 28g
- Fat: 41g
- Carbohydrates: 133g

Portobello Stuffed With Quinoa

Servings: 4
Preparation time: 20 minutes
Cook time: 25 minutes

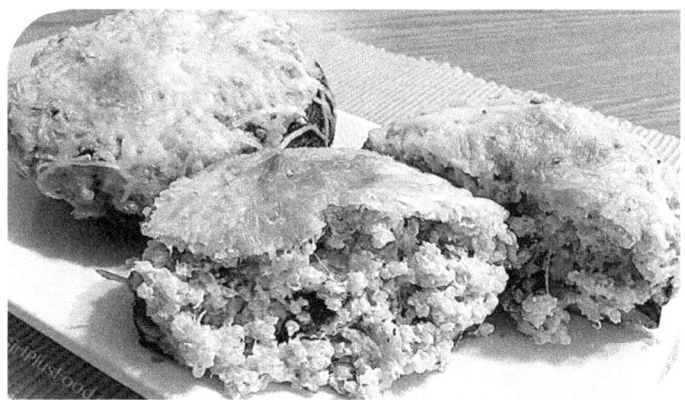

Ingredients

- 4 medium-sized Portobello mushrooms
- 2 cups cooked quinoa
- 1 ½ cups Italian tomato sauce or pizza sauce
- 1 sliced tomato (4 slices)
- 1 cup vegan mozzarella cheese (grated)
- Fresh basil leaves
- To marinate the portobello
- 6 tbsp soy sauce
- 1 tbsp garlic powder

Steps to Cook

1. Clean the mushrooms with a cloth, remove the stem and with the help of a spoon remove the inside, scraping little by little until everything is removed.
2. In a large container, place the soy sauce and garlic powder. In that same container, add the mushrooms and make sure that the sauce and garlic powder mixture comes in contact with all the mushrooms. Let marinate for 15 minutes.
3. Prepare the quinoa using vegetable broth instead of water for added flavor. When ready let it rest.
4. In a frying pan over medium high heat add a few drops of olive oil. When it is hot, place a portobello and cook on each side until they are lightly browned. Repeat the operation with each mushroom and remove from the heat.
5. Preheat oven to 350^0F. Place the mushrooms on a lightly oiled baking sheet, with the inside of the mushrooms facing up. Fill each with quinoa and then add a layer of tomato sauce and a slice of tomato for each portobello. Cook for 10 minutes. If you do not have an oven you can do it in a toaster oven or in a pan with a lid. Serve with fresh basil and additional tomato sauce if you like.

Nutritional Information:

- Calorie: 408.2
- Protein: 26.9g
- Fat: 18.2g
- Carbohydrates: 73.1g

Barbecue Vegan Burritos

Servings: 2
Preparation time: 10 minutes
Cook time: 20 minutes

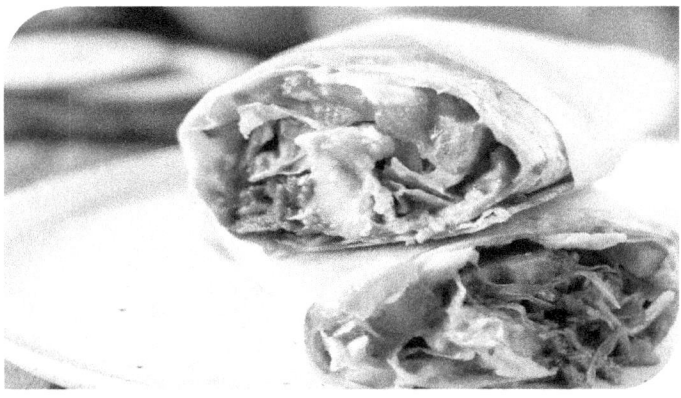

Ingredients

- ½ lb. tempeh
- 1 tablespoon of oil
- ¼ cup of barbecue sauce
- 2 medium diced tomatoes
- ½ red onion, chopped
- 1 large diced avocado
- 1 tbsp jalapeño
- A bunch of chopped coriander
- The juice of half a lime
- a pinch of salt
- 4 large tortillas mine
- 3 ½ oz. of cut lettuce

Steps to Cook

1. Cut the tempeh into 8 sheets. If your tempeh is bitter, boil or steam it for 15 minutes. This helps improve texture as well. Dry with a cloth.
2. Heat a large skillet over medium-high heat and add the oil. Once it is hot, add the tempeh. Fry, turning, until golden brown on both sides.
3. Brush with barbecue sauce, turn it over and fry for a minute to caramelize. Brush the other side with sauce and flip once more. Fry 1 minute more to caramelize this side as well. Remove from the heat and if you have barbecue sauce, add it to the tempeh.
4. In a bowl combine the tomato, onion, avocado, coriander, jalapeño, salt and lime.
5. Fill each tortilla with a little lettuce, salad and two slices of the tempeh. Fold the omelette.

Nutritional Information:

- Calorie: 404
- Protein: 12g
- Fat: 18g
- Carbohydrates: 49g

Oriental Style Vegetables

Servings: 2
Preparation time: 5 minutes
Cook time: 5 minutes

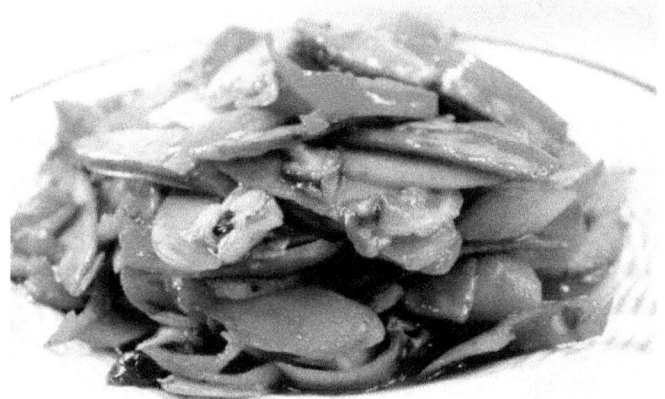

Ingredients

- 1 ½ oz. mushrooms
- A piece of cabbage or Chinese cabbage
- 1 carrot
- Half an onion
- 1 piece of red, green, yellow bell pepper
- 1 clove garlic
- Salt to taste
- Soy sauce to taste
- A splash of dry white wine
- ¼ cup of soft olive oil

Steps to Cook

1. Clean and chop all the ingredients and cut them into strips, like a thick julienne.
2. In a deep-frying pan or better a wok, heat the oil over the fire. When it is very hot put all the chopped vegetables at the same time with the crushed garlic.
3. Fry without stopping stirring a couple of minutes, salt (carefully because you will add soy later) and add the wine. While continuing to stir keep on the fire another couple of minutes.
4. As soon as the alcohol evaporates, you must remove the dish from the heat. The vegetables must be whole, al dente. When serving, sprinkle with a little soy sauce and sprinkle with sesame seeds.

Nutritional Information:

- Calorie: 24.7
- Protein: 1g
- Fat: 0g
- Carbohydrates: 5g

Jamaican Flower Tacos

Servings: 6
Preparation time: 10 minutes
Cook time: 10 minutes

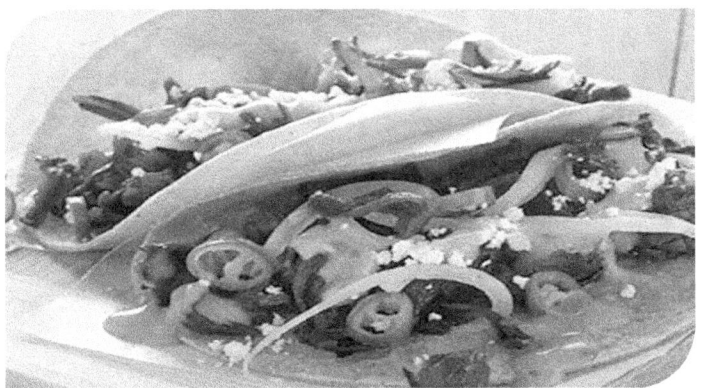

Ingredients

- 1 tablespoon avocado oil or another neutral flavor
- ½ cup chopped onion
- 2 cups Jamaica flower already boiled and chopped
- 1 jalapeño or serrano pepper
- salt to taste
- At your service
- 12 corn tortillas
- 2 avocados or guacamole

Steps to Cook

1. To prepare it, make Jamaica water as usual. Rinse the flower and drain it very well. In a separate frying pan put the oil and the chopped onion to brown.
2. While the Jamaica is minced or put it in the food processor to make it into smaller pieces. This step is important especially if the flower comes very whole.
3. When the onion is golden brown put the Jamaica and a jalapeño or serrano pepper. I put it in large pieces so that I can remove it later if someone doesn't want it.
4. When the flower feels well dry, it means that it is done, add a little salt and that's it..

Nutritional Information:

- Calorie: 200
- Protein: 3g
- Fat: 12g
- Carbohydrates: 24g

Vegan Burrito In Bowl

Servings: 4
Preparation time: 5 minutes
Cook time: 15 minutes

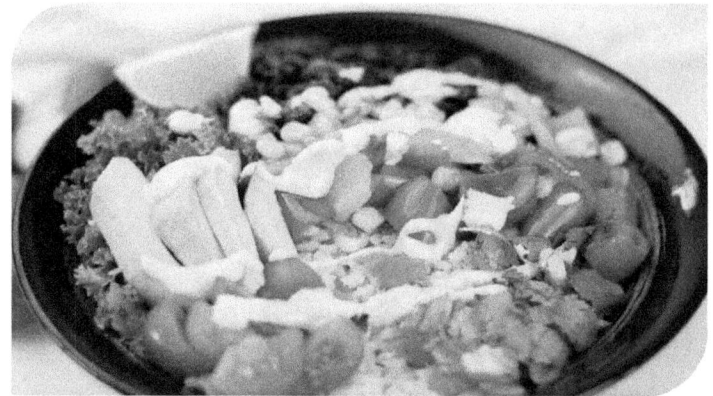

Ingredients

For the coriander and lime sauce:
- 2 oz. of raw cashew nuts
- ½ cup of water
- 1 ½ oz. of fresh coriander
- The juice of a lime
- 1 teaspoon salt

For the vegan burrito in bowl:
- 2 tbsp of olive oil
- Half a medium onion
- 2 garlic cloves, minced
- ½ lb. of rice
- 1 cup of vegetable stock
- ¾ cup crushed tomato
- ½ tsp of cumin
- ½ tsp of ground chili
- 1 tbsp of oregano
- 1 tsp salt
- Pepper to taste
- 1 red bell pepper

Steps to Cook

1. For the coriander and lime sauce
2. Drain the cashews and add them with the other ingredients to a blender or food processor. Process until obtaining a creamy sauce. Transfer to the fridge to thicken.
3. For the vegan burrito in bowl
4. Heat a pot over medium-high heat. Add 1 tablespoon of oil and sauté the onion and garlic. Add the rice, broth or water, crushed tomato, cumin, ground chili, oregano, salt and pepper and bring to a boil. Lower the heat and cook until the rice is soft and the liquid has been absorbed. Add a little more broth or water if it seems to be drying.
5. Meanwhile heat a grill pan (or a regular skillet if you use canned corn) over medium-high heat. Brush the corn and bell pepper with 1 tablespoon of oil and add salt. Grill (or fry) until soft and grilled. Once it has cooled down enough, cut the pepper into squares and remove the cob.
6. Once the rice is ready, add the beans and put together the bowls. Start with the rice and bean mixture and top with the roasted vegetables, cherry tomatoes, and avocado. Garnish with coriander and

- 1 ear of corn leafless
- ½ lb. of cooked beans
- ½ lb. of cooked beans
- 2 of cherry tomatoes
- 1 avocado, cut

lime if you like and serve with the coriander and lime sauce.

Nutritional Information:

- Calorie: 580
- Protein: 16.5g
- Fat: 22.5g
- Carbohydrates: 85g

Vegetable Stuffed Courgettes

Servings: 3
Preparation time: 15 minutes
Cook time: 45-60 minutes

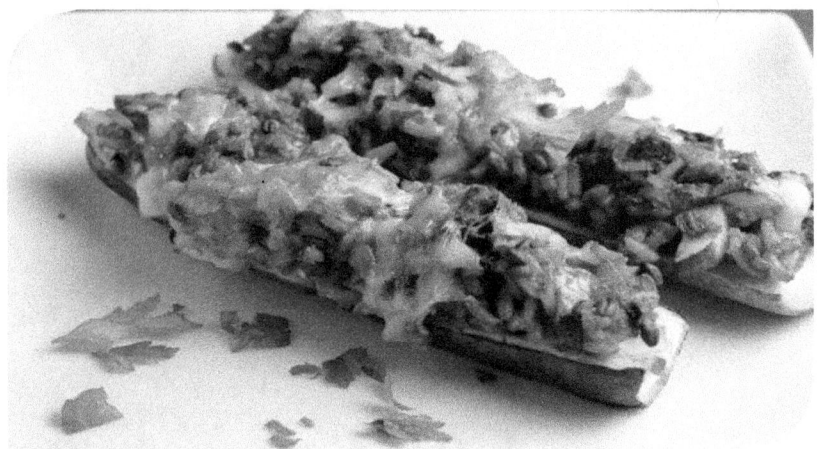

Ingredients

- 2 small red onions
- 2 small brown peppers
- 2 small round zucchinis
- 3 garlic cloves, minced
- ½ lb. of chopped mushrooms
- 1 carrot, chopped
- 2 tsp of paprika
- 2 tsp dried marjoram
- 1 tsp dried thyme
- ½ lb. of cooked lentils
- ½ cup dried tomato
- 1 tsp of salt
- Pepper

Steps to Cook

1. Preheat the oven to 400°F. Cut the tops of the vegetables and scoop out the insides with a spoon. Chop the insides of the zucchini and onions.
2. Heat a frying pan over medium high heat and add the inside of the onions, garlic and a splash of water. Once poached, add the mushrooms and fry until golden. Add the carrot and the inside of the zucchini. Fry until soft and the liquid has evaporated.
3. Add the paprika and herbs and fry for a few seconds to release the aroma. Add the lentils, fried tomato, salt and pepper and cook for a few minutes so that the flavors mix. Season the interiors of the empty vegetables and fill with the lentils. Place them on a tray and return their lids. Bake 45 to 60 minutes or until easily pricked with a knife. Check them out from time to time and if the lids start to burn.

Nutritional Information:

- Calorie: 237.1
- Protein: 12.5g
- Fat: 7.4g
- Carbohydrates: 33g

Vegan Ceviche

Servings: 2
Preparation time: 10 minutes

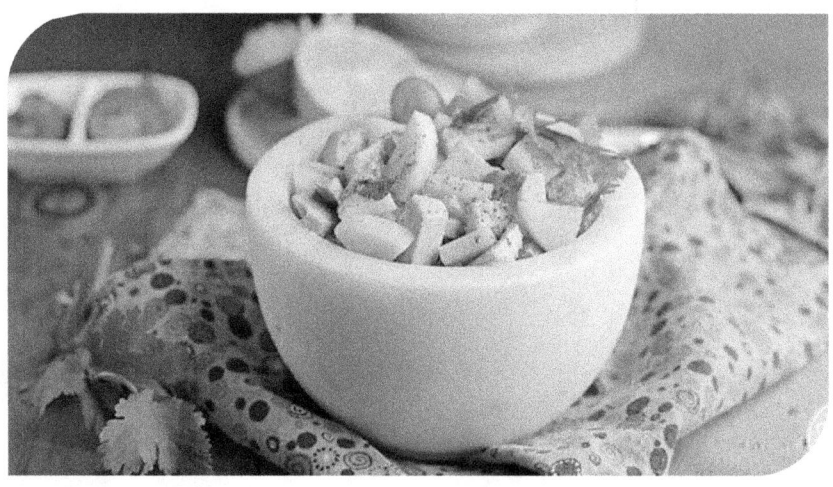

Ingredients

- 1 can of 1 lb. of canned hearts of palm (14 oz), chopped and without the liquid
- 2 chopped tomatoes
- ½ red onion, chopped
- 2 tablespoons chopped parsley or coriander
- 2 tbsp lemon juice
- 2 tbsp of nori seaweed flakes
- ¼ tsp of salt

Steps to Cook

1. Mix all the ingredients in a container until they are well integrated.
2. Ceviche can be eaten immediately, but the ideal is to let it rest covered in the fridge for at least 1 hour, so it will have a more intense flavor.
3. You can keep it in an airtight container in the fridge for 1 or 2 days.

Nutritional Information:

- Calorie: 262.7
- Protein: 4.7g
- Fat: 20.9g
- Carbohydrates: 18.3g

Servings: 4

Pico Of Gallo

Preparation time: 15 minutes

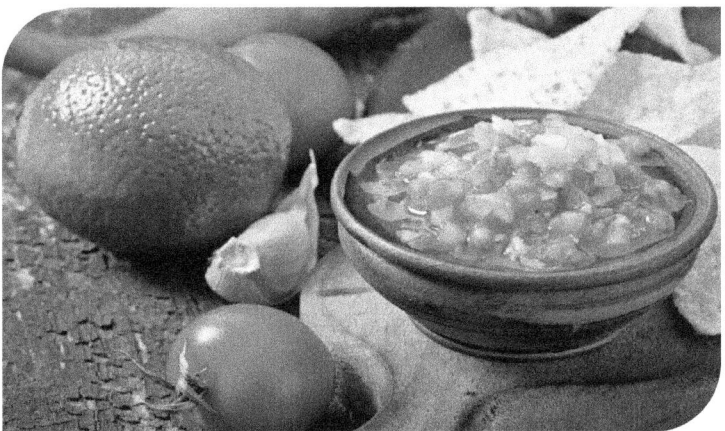

Ingredients

- 1 piece of mango
- 1 jalapeño pepper
- 1 tomato ball
- 1 white onion
- 1 jicama girl
- 1 bunch of coriander
- 1 tbsp mint leaves
- 2 lemons
- 1 teaspoon of olive oil
- 1 tbsp of piquín chili powder
- 1 tbsp of salt
- 1 tsp of pepper
- Blue tortilla chips to taste

Steps to Cook

1. On a medium board, chop the mango, tomato, onion, chili and jicama.
2. Put everything in a bowl and reserve.
3. Add the lemon juice and olive oil.
4. Chop the coriander and peppermint.
5. Season with salt and pepper.

Nutritional Information:

- Calorie: 11
- Protein: 0.4g
- Fat: 0.1g
- Carbohydrates: 2.5g

Curled Lentils With Spinach

Servings: 4

Preparation time: 10 minutes

Cook time: 30-35 minutes

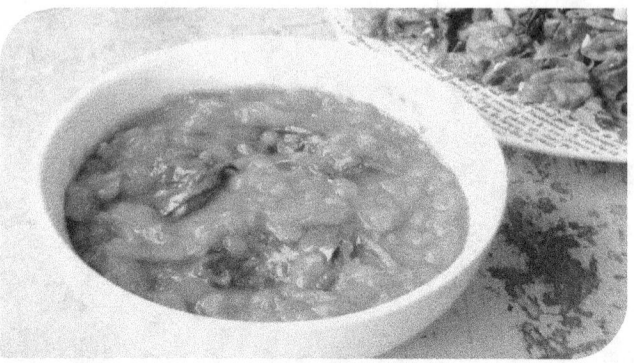

Ingredients

- 2 tbsp of olive oil
- 1 ½ cups chopped onion
- 1 cup chopped celery
- 1 cup peeled carrots
- 3 garlic cloves, minced
- 1 tbsp of curry powder
- 1 tbsp fresh ginger
- 1 tsp of ground cumin
- 1 bay leaf
- ¼ tsp dry red pepper
- 9 ½ cups of water
- 16 ounces dried lentils
- 6 oz spinach leaves
- ½ cup fresh coriander

Steps to Cook

1. Heat the oil in a large saucepan over medium heat.
2. Add onion, celery, carrots, garlic, and sauté for 10 minutes until golden.
3. Add the curry powder, ginger, cumin, dried bay leaves, and crushed red pepper.
4. Add 9 ½ cups of water, dried lentils and bring to a boil.
5. Reduce heat to medium-low heat and cook until lentils are tender.
6. If you like the fine broth, add more water (1/2 cup) and cook for about 25 minutes.
7. Add the spinach and coriander; cooking them for approximately 5 more minutes.
8. Add salt and pepper to taste.

Nutritional Information:

- Calorie: 537
- Protein: 33.6g
- Fat: 8.8g
- Carbohydrates: 83.2g

Peruvian Sautéed Loin

Servings: 4
Preparation time: 5 minutes
Cook time: 5 minutes

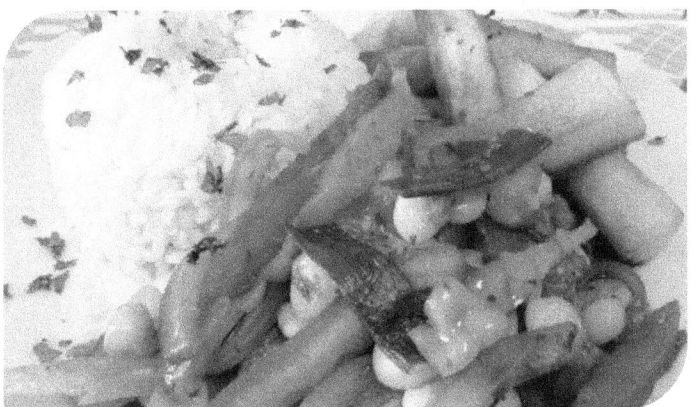

Ingredients

- 4 lbs. white potato
- 3 ½ oz. soy meat
- 3 tomatoes
- 1 small of green pepper
- 1 fresh garlic
- 3 oz. peas
- 3 oz. green beans
- 1 piece of ginger
- 2 carrots, diced
- ½ cup of water
- 1 teaspoon of cumin
- 2 bay leaves
- 2 oregano leaves
- Salt, pepper to taste

Steps to Cook

1. Cut the potatoes long and fry them.
2. If you use ground soybean meat, rehydrate it in boiled water.
3. In a saucepan, fry the ginger for about a minute.
4. Add the bell pepper, bay leaf and a little oregano, cumin and pepper.
5. Add the washed soybeans, peas, and salt.
6. Finally pour the water and boil until the vegetables are cooked.
7. Add the sliced tomatoes and the fried potato.
8. Serve with white rice.

Nutritional Information:

- Calorie: 175.9
- Protein: 5.8g
- Fat: 9.1g
- Carbohydrates: 19.6g

Chickpea And Avocado Sandwich

Servings: 2
Preparation time: 5 minutes

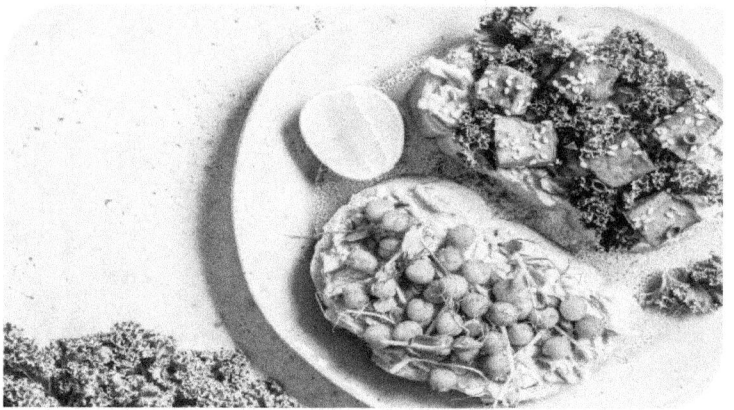

Ingredients

- 1 cup cooked chickpeas
- 1 medium avocado
- 1 small onion
- 2 tablespoons fresh coriander or mint leaves
- 2 butter spoons
- 2 slices of bread
- Juice of 1 lemon
- Salt and pepper

Steps to Cook

1. To start with the preparation of this delicious sandwich, the first thing you should do is peel and chop the onion and avocado very well.
2. If you do not have this food you can use cucumber.
3. Now puree the cooked chickpeas and add the chopped onion, coriander (or mint leaves), chopped avocado, lemon juice, salt and pepper.
4. Mix all these elements very well until achieving a good consistency.

Nutritional Information:

- Calorie: 695
- Protein: 16.2g
- Fat: 15.7g
- Carbohydrates: 122.1g

Mediterranean Nachos

Servings: 4
Preparation time: 5 minutes
Cooking time: 30 minutes

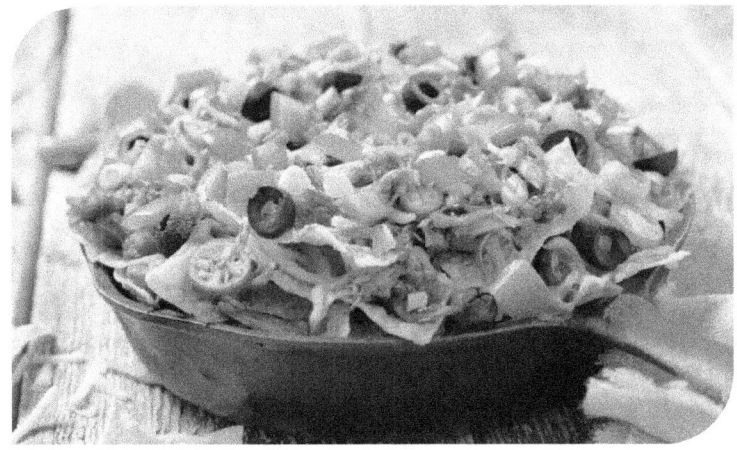

Ingredients

- 3 ½ oz. cooked corn kernels
- ½ lb. of Mexican chips
- 3 oz. black olives
- 1 ½ oz. of mimolette cheese
- 1 lbs. crushed tomato or pot sauce
- 12 cherry or cherry tomatoes
- 1 ½ oz. soft Cantal cheese

Steps to Cook

1. Cut the black olives in half.
2. Wash the cherry or cherry tomatoes and cut them in half lengthwise.
3. Grate the two cheeses. If you don't get any of them, you can use another cheese to grate, such as Parmesan.
4. Preheat the oven to 360°F and distribute the nachos in a bowl.
5. Top with the crushed tomato sauce and pour over the cooked corn kernels.
6. Add the black olives and tomatoes.
7. Spread the cheeses over the top and bake for 8 to 10 minutes, or until the cheese has melted.

Nutritional Information:

- Calorie: 253
- Protein: 12g
- Fat: 12g
- Carbohydrates: 23g

Vegetarian Vegetable Lasagna

Servings: 2
Preparation time: 20 minutes
Cooking time: 45 minutes

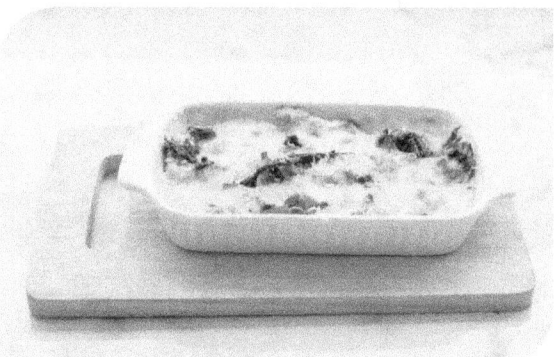

Ingredients

- 1 eggplant
- 2 zucchinis
- 1 onion
- 2 garlic
- 2 ½ cup of tomato paste
- 1 egg
- 1 tbsp of basil
- 1 cup of mozzarella cheese
- 1 cup of Parmesan cheese
- Salt
- pepper and olive oil

Steps to Cook

1. Preheat the oven to 360ºF. In a frying pan add a drizzle of olive oil, add the previously chopped onion and garlic, let them brown for a few minutes and add the tomato paste and basil, stir, add salt and pepper if necessary.
2. Meanwhile, cut the eggplant and zucchini lengthwise into medium strips, which are neither too thick nor too thin, in a pan, add another teaspoon of oil and put the strips of the vegetables so that they "roast" for both sides, remove and reserve.
3. In another container mix the cheeses and add the egg, stir until well mixed, finally the container that you are going to use to cook the lasagna should be smeared with margarine so that the ingredients are not going to stick.
4. Place a layer of the vegetables, then a layer of the sauce and a layer of cheese, until the container is full, but do not leave it completely overflowing, at the end add a layer of mozzarella cheese, take to the oven for 30 minutes or until you see the cheese a little gratin.

Nutritional Information:

- Calorie: 360
- Protein: 23g
- Fat: 11g
- Carbohydrates: 45g

- Calorie: 360
- Protein: 23g
- Fat: 11g
- Carbohydrates: 45g

Vegetarian Pizza

Servings: 2
Preparation time: 10 minutes
Cooking time: 15 minutes

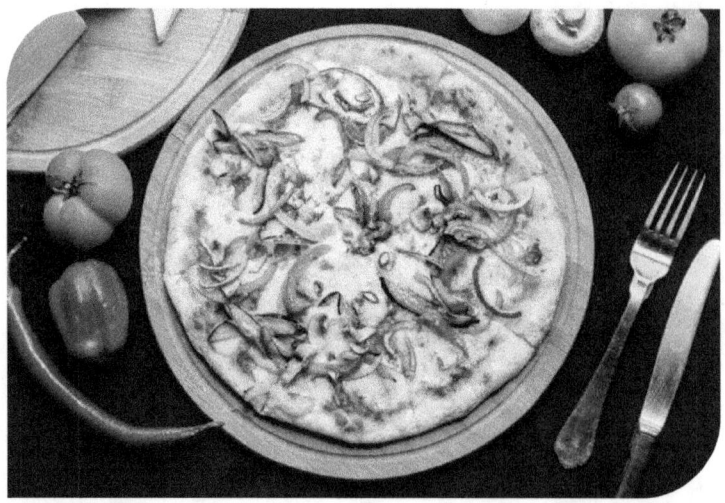

Ingredients

- pre ready pizza dough
- 1 eggplant
- 1 zucchini
- 1 red bell pepper
- 1 green paprika
- 1 ½ oz. leek
- 3 oz. onion
- 1 tbsp of capers
- tomato sauce or tomato paste
- ½ lb. grated mozzarella cheese
- olive oil and salt

Steps to Cook

1. pre heat the oven to 360°F, meanwhile wash the vegetables and cut them into small squares, in a frying pan add a jet of oil and sauté all the vegetables (without the capers) until al dente.
2. On the tray that you prepare the pizza and it will enter the oven, arrange the dough already ready, spread a layer of tomato sauce or tomato paste without reaching the edges, sprinkle the mozzarella cheese, distribute the already cooked vegetables and finally capers.
3. Bake for 15 minutes or until batter is golden brown and cheese is melted.

Nutritional Information:

- Calorie: 280
- Protein: 11g
- Fat: 9g
- Carbohydrates: 39g

Sweet Potatoes Stuffed With Black Beans

Servings: 2
Preparation time: 5 minutes
Cooking time: 15-20 minutes

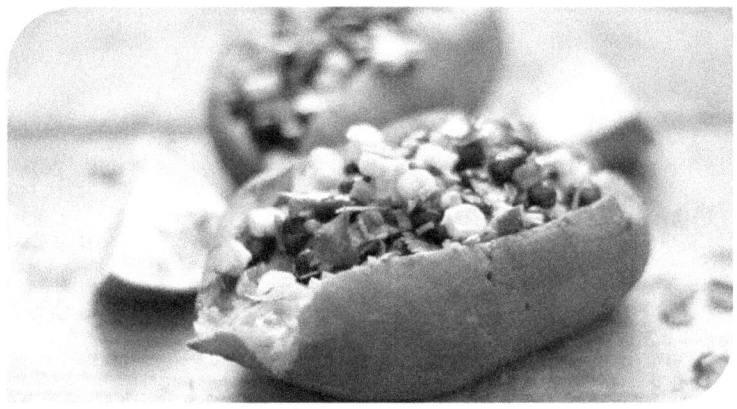

Ingredients

- 2 sweet potatoes
- 1 cup black beans, cooked
- ½ jalapeño pepper
- ¼ red onion, minced
- 2 tomatillos, minced
- ¼ cup coriander
- 1 garlic clove
- ½ lemon juice
- Salt and pepper
- Indian walnut cream

Steps to Cook

1. Steam the sweet potatoes until soft. Reserve and let them cool.
2. While the sweet potatoes are cooking, mix the beans, the tomatillos, the onion, the garlic, the jalapeño and the coriander. Add the lemon zest and juice. Season and reserve in the refrigerator.
3. When serving, the sweet potatoes are cut in half.
4. Place the sweet potatoes and distribute the filling between the two.
5. Decorate with Indian walnut cream and a few coriander leaves to serve.

Nutritional Information:

- Calorie: 261.5
- Protein: 10.2g
- Fat: 3.9g
- Carbohydrates: 46.7g

Chapter 6

Snacks & Sides

Tlacoyos Of Beans With Nopales Stew

Servings: 8
Preparation time: 5 minutes
Cooking time: 30 minutes

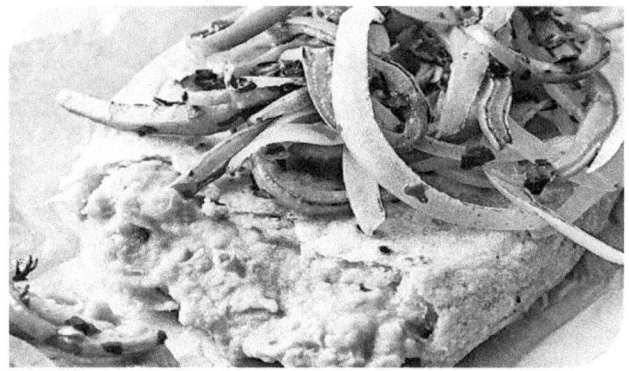

Ingredients

- 8 bean Tlacoyos
- 1 sliced onion
- 3 large nopales cut into strips
- 1 tbsp of oregano
- 2 tbsp of white vinegar
- 2 tbsp of oil
- 5 green tomatoes
- 2 serrano peppers
- 1 clove garlic
- 1 small bunch of coriander

Steps to Cook

1. Place the tomatoes, chili and garlic in aluminum foil, close well and bake at 200° C for 30 minutes.
2. Blend the entire content with the coriander; add a little water or chicken broth if necessary. Strain the sauce and reserve.
3. Cook the nopales in a pot with water, salt and vinegar. When they are almost cooked, strain them and rinse with cold water to cut the slime.
4. Heat a large skillet with the oil, grill the onion until lightly browned; then add the nopales and oregano. Cook for a few minutes; salt pepper.
5. Roast the Tlacoyos on a comal with a little oil, serve accompany with the sauce.

Nutritional Information:

- Calorie: 261
- Protein: 9.5g
- Fat: 8.6g
- Carbohydrates: 38g

Vegan & Gluten-Free Cookies Of Walnut And Blueberries

Servings: 8
Preparation time: 5 minutes
Cooking time: 20 minutes

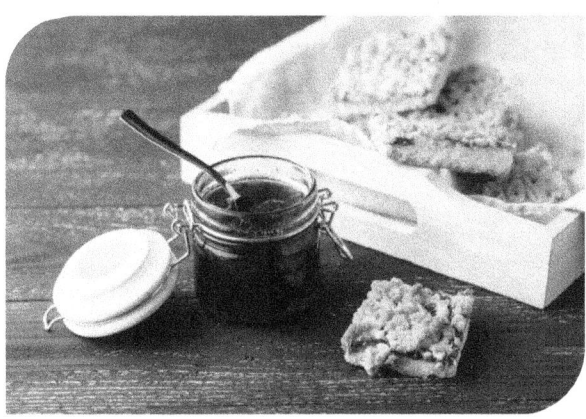

Ingredients

- 1 cup gluten-free flour
- ¾ tbsp baking powder
- ½ cup crushed nuts
- ¼ cup grated coconut
- ¼ cup muscovado sugar
- ¼ cup unrefined coconut oil
- 2 tbsp of coconut milk
- 1 tbsp of vanilla extract
- 2 tbsp blueberries

Steps to Cook

1. Preheat oven for 10 minutes at 350°F
2. In a large bowl mix the dry ingredients: flour, crushed walnuts, baking powder and grated coconut. Reserve.
3. In a bowl mix the following ingredients: sugar, coconut oil, coconut milk and vanilla extract.
4. Add the liquid mixture to the dry until it forms a dough. Add the blueberries and incorporate them into the dough.
5. Divide the dough into 8 portions and shape into a cookie. It doesn't have to be perfect. Place on a tray with a little muddy coconut oil so they do not stick.
6. Bake at 3500F for 20 minutes. Remove from the oven and let cool for 10 to 15 minutes.

Nutritional Information:

- Calorie: 261
- Protein: 9.5g
- Fat: 8.6g
- Carbohydrates: 38g

Vegan Sushi

Servings: 4

Preparation time: 1h

Cooking time: 15 minutes

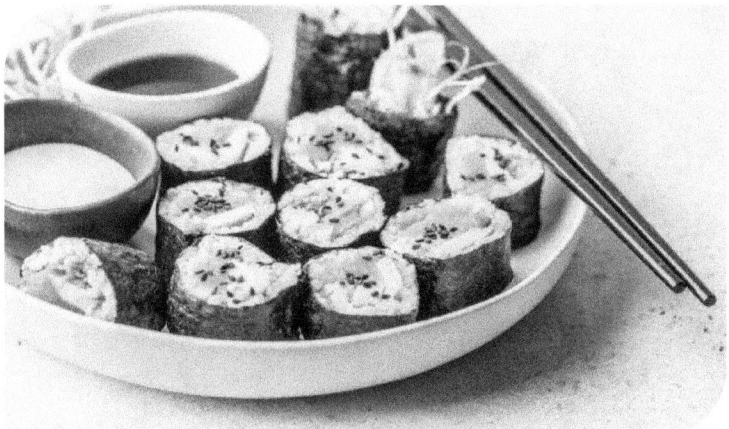

Ingredients

Rice rolls:

- ½ lb. sushi rice
- 2 tbsp vinegar
- 1 package nori seaweed
- 1 bamboo mat

Filling:

- 1 mango
- 1 avocado
- 1 cucumber
- 1 bell pepper
- 1 tempeh
- soy sauce or tamari

Steps to Cook

Cooking rice:

1. First bring the water to a boil and then add the rice. Simmer and cover the saucepan, but not completely. After 15 minutes, add the rice in a bowl
2. Once it is cooked, add the vinegar and stir gently with a wooden spoon.

Sushi:

3. If you want the roll to be covered in sesame seeds, spread them over the rice. Cover the mat with plastic wrap and place the seaweed with rice in the following way: that the rice is in contact with the plastic wrap and the seaweed on top. Place a third of the end of the filling ingredients and roll with the help of the mat and plastic wrap.

Nutritional Information:

- Calorie: 476
- Protein: 14.3g
- Fat: 12.9g
- Carbohydrates: 70.9g

Japanese Omelette Rice

Servings: 2

Preparation time: 5 minutes

Cooking time: 20-25 minutes

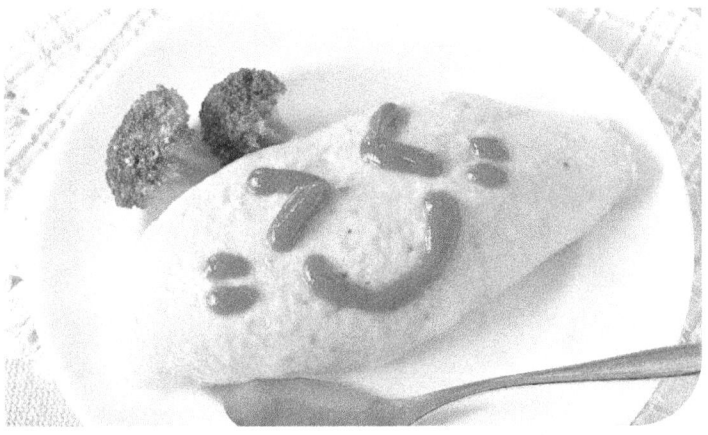

Ingredients

- ½ cup of cooked white rice
- 2 tbsp of vegetable oil
- 1 cup green bell peppers
- 1 cup red or yellow bell peppers
- 1 cup onion, chopped
- 2 tbsp of tomato sauce
- 1 large egg
- 2 tbsp of egg white
- 2 tsp of salt

Steps to Cook

1. Heat a wok with a tablespoon of vegetable oil. Fry the onion. Then add the peppers and 1 tsp of salt. Stir-fry until most of the water has evaporated. Now add the cooked rice and the tomato sauce. Stir until well incorporated into the vegetables. Reserve.
2. In another bowl, beat together the large egg, egg white and 1 tsp of salt. Heat a skillet with 1 tbsp of vegetable oil. When it is hot enough, pour the egg mixture you have just prepared there. Make sure the mixture covers the entire pan. When the omelette is almost ready, add the fried rice mixture that you had reserved. Fold the tortilla over the rice, wrapping it. When you see that everything is well cooked, transfer a plate and serve.

Nutritional Information:

- Calorie: 390
- Protein: 22.1g
- Fat: 9.2g
- Carbohydrates: 54.1g

Swiss-Style Potato And Onion Omelette

Servings: 4

Preparation time: 5 minutes

Cooking time: 20-25 minutes

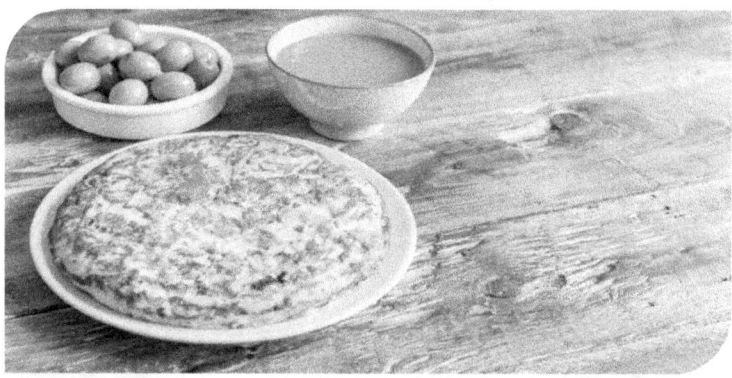

Ingredients

- 4 medium potatoes
- 1 large onion
- Sunflower oil
- Butter
- Pepper
- Salt

Steps to Cook

1. Peel the potatoes and cook them in a pot with boiling water for 10 minutes. When removed from the pot, the potatoes must be semi-raw. Let them cool.
2. Grate them with a traditional cheese grater. Season with salt and a pinch of black pepper.
3. Peel the onion and cut it into thin slices.
4. Sauté it in a frying pan with a splash of oil, over medium heat, until the onion is tender and golden. Place the grated potato and the cooked onion in a bowl and mix.
5. In a medium skillet pour the contents of the bowl, and crush the mixture with the help of a fork to shape it into an omelette. Cook for 10 to 12 minutes on each side over low heat.

Nutritional Information:

- Calorie: 361
- Protein: 22g
- Fat: 22g
- Carbohydrates: 18g

Potato, Ginger And Onion Tortilla

Servings: 2
Preparation time: 5 minutes
Cooking time: 15 minutes

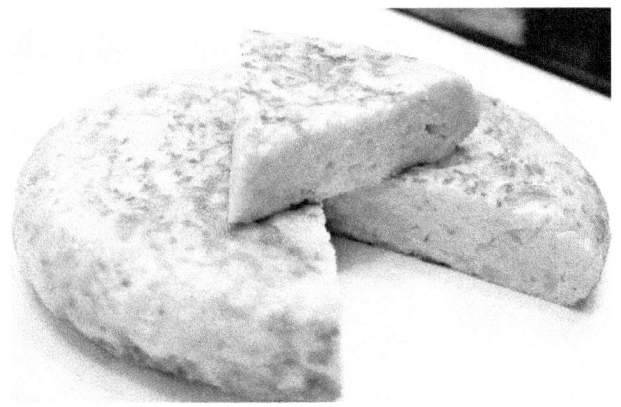

Ingredients

- 7 oz. of potato
- 1 clove garlic
- 1 tbsp grated ginger
- 7 oz. of onion
- 3 eggs
- Salt
- pepper and olive oil

Steps to Cook

1. Peel the shovels and cut them into small cubes, boil them in water with a pinch of salt until they soften, turn off and reserve.
2. On the other hand, beat the eggs and season with salt and pepper to taste and reserve. Cut the onions in julienne strips and sauté them in a frying pan with a drizzle of olive oil, also add the crushed garlic and ginger, stir well and add the ready-made potatoes.
3. Add the egg and stir well so that all the ingredients are integrated into the egg, over low heat let the tortilla curdle on one side and then turn it until it is dry on both sides.

Nutritional Information:

- Calorie: 233
- Protein: 8g
- Fat: 6g
- Carbohydrates: 39g

Lentil And Vegetable Burger

Servings: 2
Preparation time: 5 minutes
Cooking time: 30 minutes

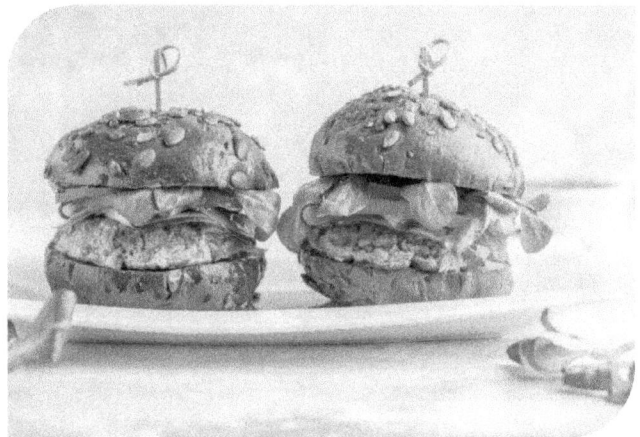

Ingredients

- ½ lb. of lentils
- 4 tbsp of breadcrumb
- 1 onion
- 5 mushrooms
- 2 garlic
- 1 paprika
- parsley
- coriander
- cumin
- Chopped cheese
- Hamburger 'bread

Steps to Cook

1. Cook the lentils in enough water, with half an onion and with a pinch of salt, when they are soft, pass them through a processor or a blender until it is like a dough, while in the processor add a little cumin, coriander and parsley finely chopped.
2. In a frying pan, add a jet of oil and sauté the crushed garlic, the mushrooms cut into slices, the paprika and the onion cut into julienne strips, until al dente and turn off.
3. With the dough of the lentils form the burgers and put them on the grill until they brown on both sides, start to assemble the burgers, on the lentil burger put the cheese and then add the salted vegetables.

Nutritional Information:

- Calorie: 89
- Protein: 4.3g
- Fat: 0.6g
- Carbohydrates: 17.3g

Zucchini Fritters

Servings: 2
Preparation time: 5 minutes
Cooking time: 30-35 minutes

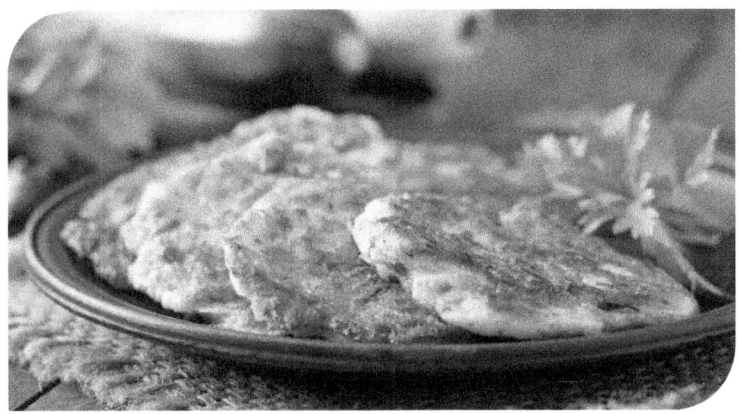

Ingredients

- 1 large zucchini
- A piece of goat cheese
- 1 egg
- ½ teaspoon onion powder
- ¼ teaspoon allspice
- 1 teaspoon salt
- ¼ tsp garlic powder

Steps to Cook

1. Grate the large zucchini to fill approximately 2 cups.
2. Once you have it, spread the salt over them and put them on a cloth to expel the water. Let it rest.
3. In a blender we put the egg together with the cheese. Mix until smooth dough remains. Add the spices and beat again.
4. Remove all the excess water that has been released. And we add the zucchini to the previous mixture. We join it very well with a wooden spoon.
5. In a tray covered with baking paper, pour 8 equal amounts of the dough.
6. Bake for 20 minutes, take them out of the oven and turn them over. Bake again for 10-15 minutes. Make sure they don't burn!

Nutritional Information:

- Calorie: 105.1
- Protein: 5.8g
- Fat: 2.8g
- Carbohydrates: 15.8g

Roasted Cauliflower

Servings: 2
Preparation time: 5 minutes
Cooking time: 15-20 minutes

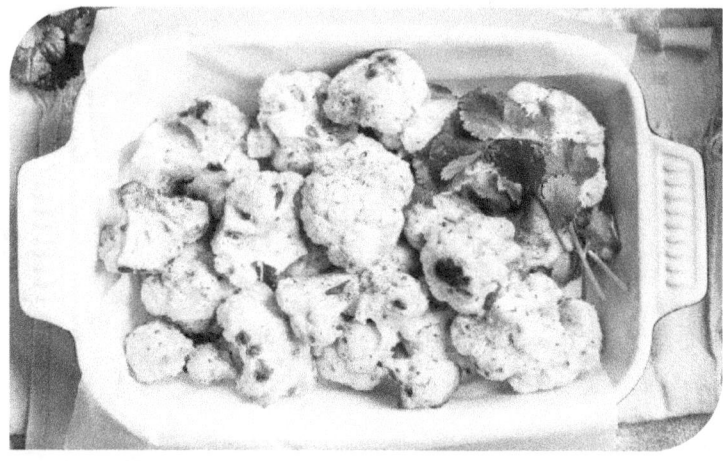

Ingredients

- 1 cauliflower
- black pepper
- Salt
- 1 teaspoon of ground cumin
- 1 tsp ground turmeric
- 1 teaspoon thyme
- ½ tsp granulated garlic
- 1 teaspoon of mustard
- 1 lemon
- fresh parsley
- extra virgin olive oil

Steps to Cook

1. Preheat the oven to 400°F. Wash the cauliflower well and dry carefully. Remove the leaves and cut the stem base slightly.
2. Heat a little olive oil in a good griddle or non-stick frying pan and cook the fillets over high heat, about 4 minutes on each side, until they are well browned. Season with salt and pepper halfway through cooking and remove to a baking tray.
3. Season with a little oil, the mustard, the lemon and all the spices. Bake for about 15-20 minutes, until lightly toasted on the outside and tender on the inside. Serve hot with chopped fresh parsley or a sauce to taste.

Nutritional Information:

- Calorie: 107
- Protein: 2.5g
- Fat: 8.9g
- Carbohydrates: 6.2g

Vegan Portobello Pizza

Servings: 4
Preparation time: 5 minutes
Cooking time: 8-10 minutes

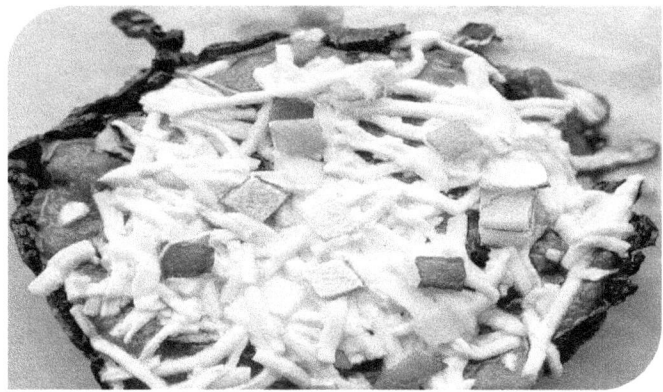

Ingredients

- 4 Units Portobello Mushroom
- 1 ¾ oz. Mozzarella Cheese
- 1 Sheet with maggi® season frying® Seasoning with Tomato and Spices
- 5 clean fresh basil leaves
- 8 Pieces Cherry tomato
- 1 pinch dried thyme
- ¼ tsp salt
- ¼ tsp black pepper

Steps to Cook

1. Clean the Portobello removing the stem, skin and membrane. Wrap two portobello in a Sheet with maggi® juicing sauce® Seasoning with Tomato and Spices, place in a frying pan over medium heat, cover and cook for 5 minutes on each side. Remove the Portobello from the sheet.
2. Place a little mozzarella cheese on the Portobello, the cherry tomatoes, basil and bake for 3 minutes or until the cheese is gratin.
3. Add a pinch of thyme and season to taste.

Nutritional Information:

- Calorie: 133.6
- Protein: 10.3g
- Fat: 6g
- Carbohydrates: 11g

Peppers Stuffed With Quinoa And Vegetables

Servings: 3

Preparation time: 15 minutes

Cooking time: 40-45 minutes

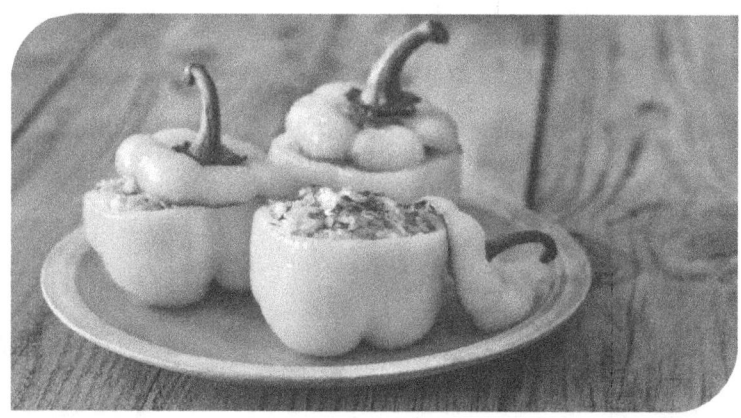

Ingredients

- 4 red peppers
- 1 bag of mixed vegetables
- 1 glass quinoa
- olive oil
- Salt
- black pepper
- oregano
- basil
- 1 tablespoon Dijon mustard

Steps to Cook

1. Wash the quinoa well and bring to a boil in a pot with two glasses of water. Leave to cook for about 15 minutes. In a frying pan with a splash of oil put the vegetables to fry well. Season with salt and pepper.
2. When you see that they soften a little, add the rest of the spices. After about 3-5minutes, add the mustard and give a few laps. Clean the peppers well on the outside and remove the hat to clean the inside of the seeds well. Put on the source of the oven with a foil to avoid dirtying.
3. Add the quinoa to the frying pan of the vegetables. Correct the point of salt and leave a few minutes that mix the flavors well. Fill the peppers with the mixture and cover with the hat. Put in the preheated oven at about 360-400°F for approximately 40-45 minutes.

Nutritional Information:

- Calorie: 340.7
- Protein: 16.8g
- Fat: 3.2g
- Carbohydrates: 65.8g

Grilled Pumpkin

Servings: 6

Preparation time: 10 minutes

Cooking time: 50 minutes

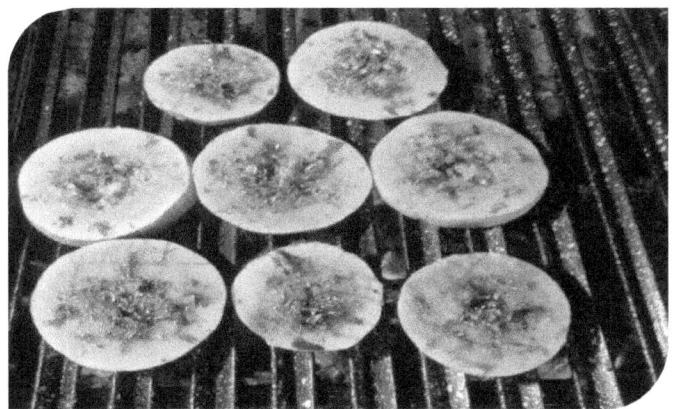

Ingredients

- 3 pumpkins (each approximately 28 oz.)
- 4 tablespoons of barbecue sauce
- 2 tablespoons of maple syrup or honey
- 4 tablespoons of dark brown sugar
- 2 tablespoons of salted butter

Steps to Cook

1. Cut each squash in half across the width. Roll ¼-inch rounded end of each half so pumpkin stays upright without wobbling. Scrape the seeds with a spoon and discard.
2. Mix barbecue sauce, maple syrup, and brown sugar in a small bowl. Divide the mixture evenly between the pumpkin halves and coat each with ½ tablespoon butter.
3. Preheat grill to medium. Put the pumpkin halves on the grill away from heat. Cook until squash is smooth and filling is golden and bubbly, about 1 hour. Remove the squash from the grill and serve immediately.

Nutritional Information:

- Calorie: 49
- Protein: 2g
- Fat: 0.2g
- Carbohydrates: 12g

Vegetarian Nuggets

Servings: 4
Preparation time: 10 minutes
Cooking time: 15-20 minutes

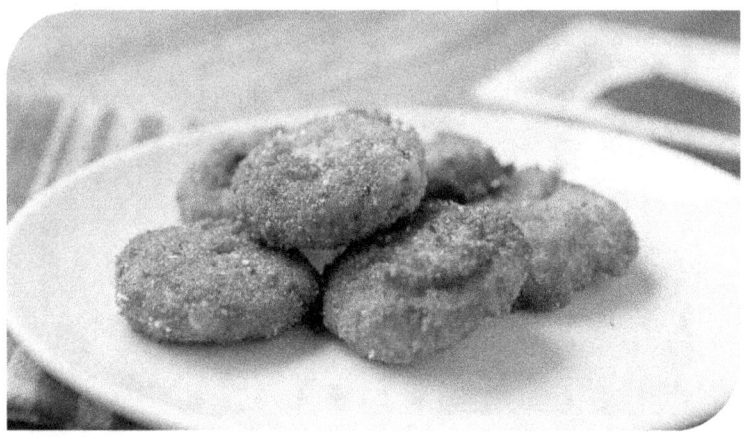

Ingredients

- 3 ½ oz. Fine textured soy
- ½ cup Water
- ¼ cup soy sauce
- 5 or 6 drops Tabasco
- Salt
- Pepper
- 3 ½ oz. breadcrumbs
- Oil for frying

Steps to Cook

1. In a bowl mix the water with the soy sauce and the tabasco, add the textured soy and leave it to soak for at least 15 minutes during which it will absorb all the liquid.
2. After that time, in another bowl, beat an egg with salt and pepper to taste, add the well-drained soybeans and 1 ½ oz. of breadcrumbs, knead until you have dough that can be compacted with your hands. If necessary, add little more breadcrumbs.
3. When you have dough that does not crumble too much, you will form pancakes with the help of your hands and fry them in abundant hot oil until they brown on both sides. Remove them to a strainer to drain and serve hot.

Nutritional Information:

- Calorie: 160
- Protein: 2g
- Fat: 5g
- Carbohydrates: 16g

Chapter 7

Desserts

Baked Onion Rings

Servings: 2-4
Preparation time: 5 minutes
Cook time: 30 minutes

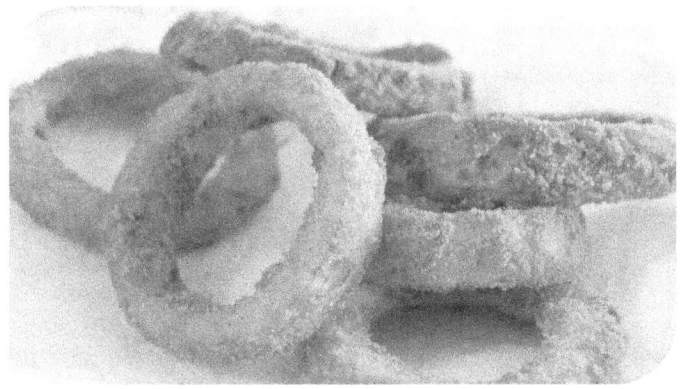

Ingredients

- 1 onion
- 4 tbsp of flour
- ¼ glass of water
- 1 tsp of apple cider vinegar
- 1 cup breadcrumbs
- 1 tbsp of olive oil
- Salt, pepper and parsley

Steps to Cook

1. Preheat the oven to 400°F. Meanwhile, cut the onion into slices not too thick so that it does not break and then separate the rings. To coat them prepare two containers. In one put the 4 tablespoons of flour, mixed with the water, the vinegar and a pinch of salt and pepper, all well mixed. In the other, the breadcrumbs with a tablespoon of oil and a little parsley. Pass the onion rings through the first container and then cover with the breadcrumbs. Place them in the tray of the greased oven. Bake until they are golden.

Nutritional Information:

- Calorie: 98
- Protein: 4g
- Fat: 1g
- Carbohydrates: 18g

Pasta Roll Stuffed with Spinach and Ricotta

Servings: 4

Preparation time: 25 minutes

Cook time: 40 minutes

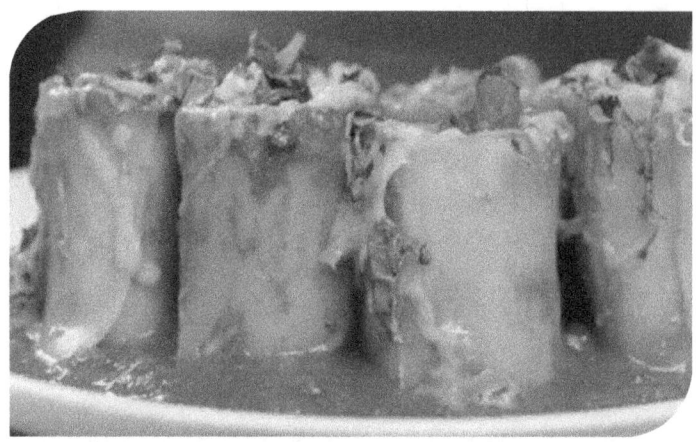

Ingredients

- 8 sheets of large lasagna
- 4 cups chopped fresh spinach
- 2 minced garlic
- ¾ lb. of ricotta
- 1 cup of grated mozzarella
- 80 g of chopped walnuts
- ½ cup grated Parmesan
- 1 egg
- 2 tbsp. chopped basil
- Salt, pepper and olive
- 2 cups tomato sauce

Steps to Cook

1. Cook pasta al dente according to package directions. Reserve.
2. In a frying pan with a little olive, sauté the garlic, add the chopped spinach and cook for 2 minutes until soft. Remove from the heat and go to a bowl.
3. Combine the bowl with the ricotta, mozzarella, Parmesan, egg, walnuts and chopped basil. Spice up.
4. Bathe the surface of an ovenproof skillet with half the tomato sauce, generously fill the sheets of pasta, roll them up and take them over the sauce. Finish with more sauce and more grated mozzarella.
5. Cover with aluminum and take to a preheated oven at 360 °F for about 25 minutes. Remove the aluminum foil and finish gratinating the cheeses for another 10 minutes.

Nutritional Information:

- Calorie: 98
- Protein: 4g
- Fat: 1g
- Carbohydrates: 18g

Potato Balls

Servings: 10

Preparation time: 40 minutes

Cook time: 10 minutes

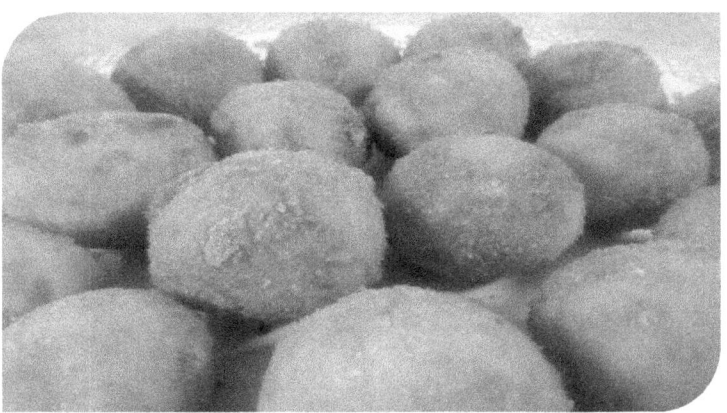

Ingredients

- 2 medium potatoes
- 3 ½ oz. butter in ointment texture
- 2 egg yolks
- flour, egg and breadcrumbs, for breading
- salt and pepper
- Olive oil

Steps to Cook

1. First, cook the potatoes. Put them in plenty of water, with a handful of salt and let them cook for about 25 minutes. Once cooked, let them temper a little and peel them. Put them in a bowl and mash well with a fork
2. Add the egg yolks, butter, pepper and a pinch of salt. Remove and integrate all the ingredients well, until there is a homogeneous mass. Then cover it and let it cool in the fridge. After time, take a teaspoon of the dough and shape it into a ball. Then go through flour, egg and breadcrumbs and reserve them on a plate, until you finish making all of them. Finally fry them. Put them in abundant olive oil but, not too strong of temperature.

Nutritional Information:

- Calorie: 181
- Protein: 6g
- Fat: 3g
- Carbohydrates: 31g

Vegetables And Tofu Skewers

Servings: 2-4
Preparation time: 5 minutes
Cook time: 10-15 minutes

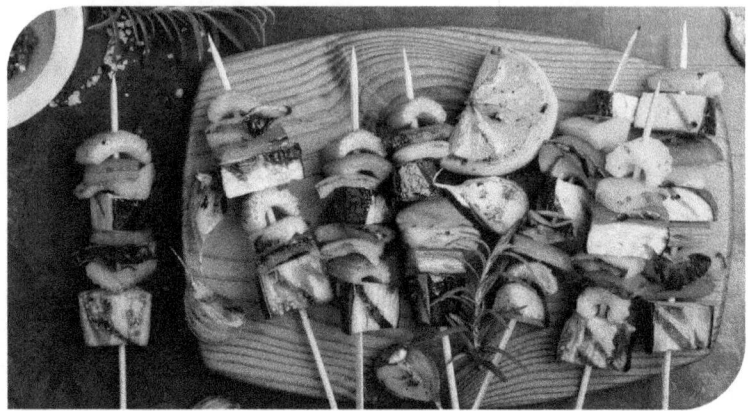

Ingredients

- Zucchini
- Cherry tomatoes
- Peppers (red and green)
- Whole fresh mushrooms
- Tofu
- Fat salt
- Pepper
- Olive oil
- Modena vinegar reduction

Steps to Cook

1. Wash the vegetables well and cut into small pieces so that they can be done well. Also cut the top to dice.
2. Then, it is placing on the sticks of the skewers.
3. Put a little olive oil on the griddle and place the skewers. Add pepper and coarse salt to taste.
4. Watch that they are made everywhere by turning them from time to time. Once ready, you can accompany them with vinegar reduction or another sauce that you like.

Nutritional Information:

- Calorie: 290
- Protein: 16g
- Fat: 9g
- Carbohydrates: 30g

Fried Banana

Servings: 04

Preparation time: 60 minutes

Cook time: 40 minutes

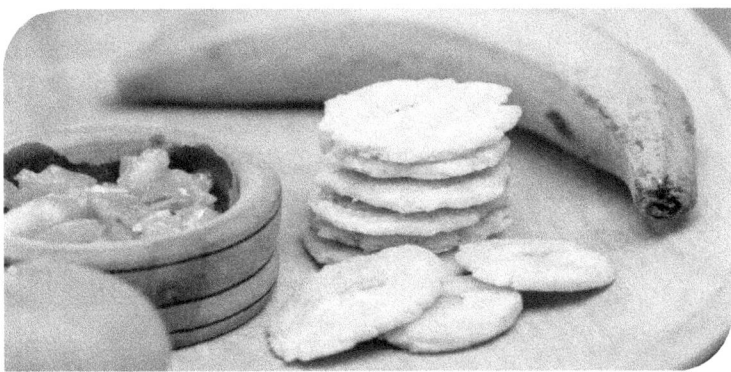

Ingredients

- 4 frying bananas
- Salt
- olive oil

Steps to Cook

1. Cut the bananas into 3-4-millimeter sheets, along them, and then separate the skin of the banana meat, using a knife. You have to remove all the green and fibrous part.
2. In a frying pan add approximately 2 millimeters of olive oil, and heat over medium heat. When the oil is hot, add the banana in batches. Let the banana of each batch fry 2 minutes on each side, until both sides are golden brown, but without passing or they will burn.
3. When the banana has browned, remove it from the pan and place it on a grid to remove the rest of the oil and add a little salt to add flavor.

Nutritional Information:

- Calorie: 378
- Protein: 4.6g
- Fat: 22g
- Carbohydrates: 44g

Chips Potatoes

Servings: 2

Preparation time: 20 minutes

Cook time: 4 minutes

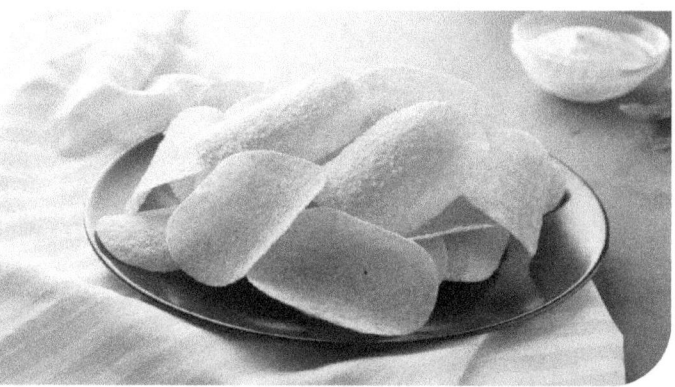

Ingredients

- 2 Potatoes
- oil. Enough to cover them completely
- Salt

Steps to Cook

1. With a peeler, peel the potatoes
2. Cut them. If you have mandolin better. If you do not have, you can cut them with the same peeler. The peeler will not give very fine cuts, which is what you need.
3. Once cut, put them in a drainer and wash them with plenty of water.
4. Drain the water from the potatoes and fry them. The oil must be very hot and it is better to do it in small batches, so that it does not get cold. While cooking, we stir them occasionally with a slotted spoon so they don't stick together and cook more evenly
5. After about 4 minutes, when you see that they are golden and with the same slotted spoon, you can see that they are crispy and remove them and place them on absorbent paper.

Nutritional Information:

- Calorie: 152
- Protein: 2g
- Fat: 9.8g
- Carbohydrates: 15g

Caramelized Onion

Servings: 2

Preparation time: 5 minutes

Cook time: 10 minutes

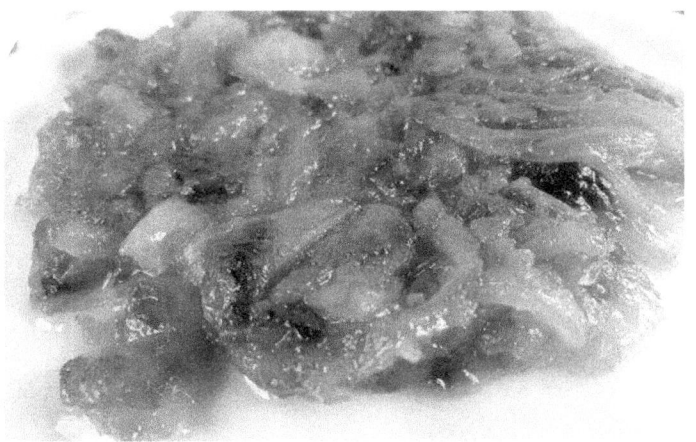

Ingredients

- An onion
- Olive oil
- A teaspoon of sugar
- A splash of vinegar

Steps to Cook

1. Cut the onion. You can cut it as you want.
2. Add a splash of oil to a pan over medium-low heat. And add the onion, with a little salt so that it begins to sweat and cook earlier.
3. Constantly stir with a wooden spoon. After about 5 minutes, add the sugar. Leave about 10 minutes more to caramelize and integrate with the onion. Continue stirring. It is important to stir because otherwise the onion is going to be toasted and that does not matter.
4. It is time to add the vinegar. Once thrown, let the liquids evaporate and voila!

Nutritional Information:

- Calorie: 152
- Protein: 2g
- Fat: 9.8g
- Carbohydrates: 15g

Watermelon Gazpacho

Servings: 2-4
Preparation time: 5 minutes

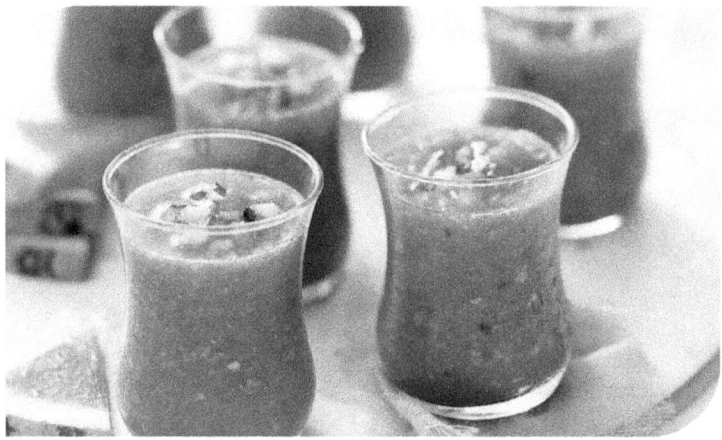

Ingredients

- 1 lb. of watermelon, without seeds
- 1 lb. of tomato
- 1 clove garlic
- Vinegar
- Water
- Extra virgin olive oil
- Salt

Steps to Cook

1. Put the garlic clove, peeled and without the central germ, the tomato, the watermelon, the vinegar, the oil and the salt, in the glass of the mixer. Crush very well, add water until the desired texture is obtained and store in the refrigerator until serving time. You can serve it with a few watermelon cubes.
2. You can prepare it with Thermomix so you don't have to peel the tomatoes and you don't have to pass it. If you do not have a very powerful mixer, peel the tomatoes, so you will not have to pass it by a Chinese in case you have any remaining skin that is always very annoying.

Nutritional Information:

- Calorie: 33
- Protein: 0.8g
- Fat: 0.4g
- Carbohydrates: 7.4g

Tofu And Chocolate Mousse

Servings: 3
Preparation time: 20 minutes
Cook time: 5-10 minutes

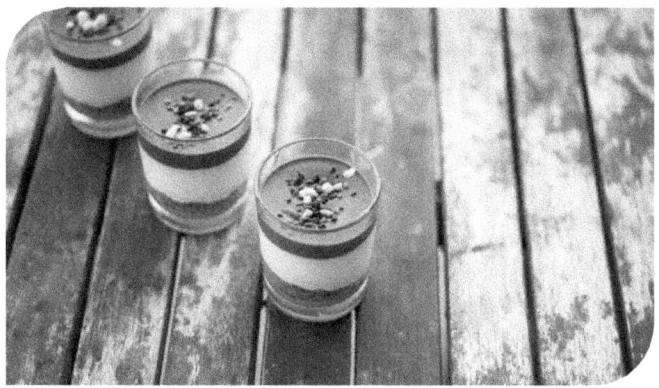

Ingredients

- 3 ½ oz. dark chocolate
- 4 oz. silky tofu at room temperature, strained
- 2 tablespoons maple syrup (can be replaced with honey, stevia, or corn syrup)

Steps to Cook

1. Melt the chocolate in the microwave, at intervals of 30 seconds, mixing between one and the other, until it is completely melted.
2. Let warm. Beat the tofu with the syrup until it is creamy. Add the chocolate and continue beating until integrated. Serve in glasses and let stand in the fridge for 2 or 3 hours before serving.
3. You can accompany it with fresh fruit, grated chocolate, nuts, etc.

Nutritional Information:

- Calorie: 109.6
- Protein: 3.4g
- Fat: 5.6g
- Carbohydrates: 11.9g

Carrot Cake

Servings: 4
Preparation time: 15 minutes
Cook time: 45 minutes

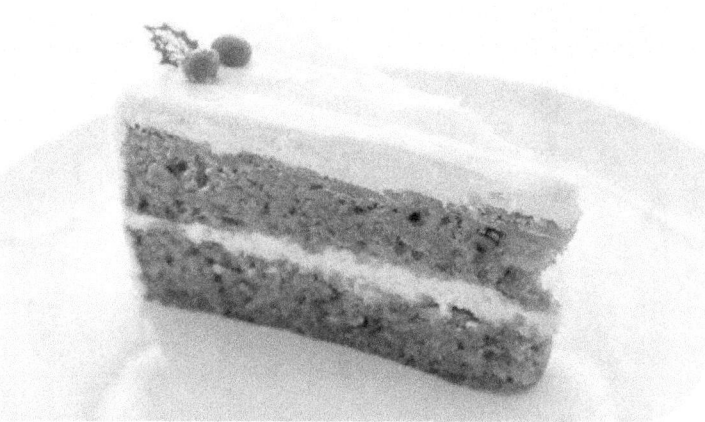

Ingredients

For the carrot cake:
- 3 cups of flour
- 2 cups of sugar
- 2 tsp. ground cinnamon
- 2 tsp. baking powder
- 1 tsp. baking soda
- 1 tsp. of salt
- 4 large eggs
- 1 ¼ cups of vegetable oil
- ¾ cup sugar-free and fat-free applesauce
- 1 tsp. vanilla extract
- 2 cups carrots, crumbled
- 1 pineapple, drained and chopped
- 1 cup chopped walnuts

For the cream cheese topping:

Steps to Cook

1. Preheat oven to 360°F and grease three 8-inch round cake pans with non-stick spray.
2. In large bowl, beat together flour, sugar, cinnamon, baking powder, baking soda, and salt.
3. In a small bowl, beat the eggs, oil, applesauce, and vanilla.
4. Add the egg mixture into the flour mixture until combined. Fold the carrots, pineapple and walnuts.
5. Evenly distribute the dough between the prepared pans and bake in the oven for about 45 minutes. Let cool.
6. For the Coverage: Place the butter and cream cheese in a bowl and beat on medium low speed until smooth and creamy, about 3 minutes. Gradually add powdered sugar. Whisk over medium until light and fluffy, scraping bowl as needed.
7. Remove the cooled cakes from their cans and place one of the layers, flat side down, on a flat plate or cake stand. Cover with ¾ cup of frosting. Put another layer of cake. Cover with ¾ cup of frosting. Place with the final layer of cake. Using a spatula,

- 1 cup unsalted butter, softened
- 1 cup cream cheese, soft
- 1 ½ cups powdered sugar
- 1 cup chopped walnuts

cover the cake with the remaining topping. Garnish with chopped walnuts along the bottom edge of the sides. Enjoy!

Nutritional Information:

- Calorie: 133.5
- Protein: 4.3g
- Fat: 3.7g
- Carbohydrates: 23.7g

Carrot And Tofu Cake

Servings: 4
Preparation time: 15 minutes
Cook time: 40 minutes

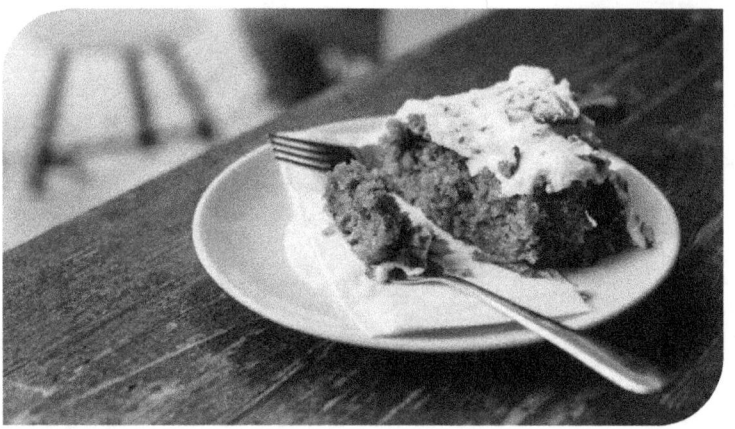

Ingredients

- ½ lb. of raw carrots, peeled and grated
- ½ lb. silky tofu
- ½ cup of sunflower oil
- ½ lb. of flour
- ½ lb. of brown sugar
- 4 tsp (one sachet) of chemical yeast
- 4 eggs
- 1 tsp of baking soda
- 1 tsp of cinnamon

Steps to Cook

1. Crush the carrots together with the oil and reserve. Sift together the dry ingredients (flour, yeast, baking soda, and cinnamon). In a large bowl beat the sugar with the eggs until they are frothy.
2. Add the tofu and continue beating to integrate. Add the carrot, mix, and then dry ingredients twice, mixing well.
3. Pour into a 24 cm mold previously greased and floured. Take to the oven preheated to 360° F for about 40 minutes, to know if the cake is ready click with a toothpick in the center, if it comes out clean it is cooked.
4. Remove from the oven, let cool in the mold and then unmold.

Nutritional Information:

- Calorie: 133.5
- Protein: 4.3g
- Fat: 3.7g
- Carbohydrates: 23.7g

Servings: 4

Preparation time: 10 minutes

Cook time: 40 minutes

Strawberry Cream Cake

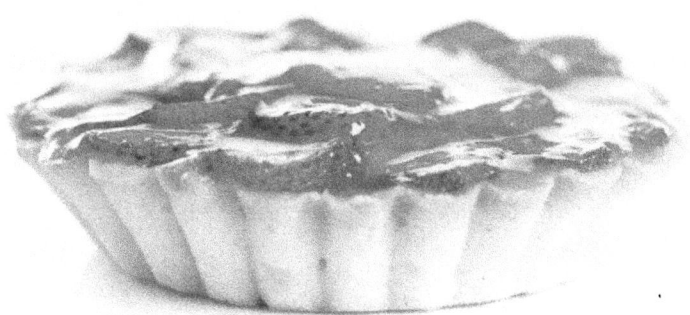

Ingredients

- 4 eggs
- 1 cup of sugar
- ¼ cup oil
- 1 cup of flour
- 1 pinch of salt
- ½ cup boiling water
- ½ tsp. vanilla extract tea
- Powdered tea
- 1 ½ teaspoon of baking soda
- ½ lb. of fresh cream
- 3 ½ oz. condensed milk
- 1 lb. strawberry

Steps to Cook

1. Separate the whites from the yolks and reserve the whites. In a bowl, beat the egg yolks with the sugar and oil. Mix the flour with the salt.
2. Add the water and wheat flour to the yolk mixture and mix. Then add the vanilla essence. Beat the egg whites.
3. Add the yeast mixture and finally the egg whites gently.
4. Grease and flour a mold with a round shape and place the mixture
5. Bake at 360°F for 40 minutes.
6. Mix the cream with condensed milk to form whipped cream.
7. Cut ½ lb. of strawberries in small cubes and add to the mixture of whipped cream Mix with the rest of the whipped cream.
8. Cover the cake with the cream and decorate.

Nutritional Information:

- Calorie: 212.5
- Protein: 2.3g
- Fat: 8.3g
- Carbohydrates: 31.9g

Quince Sweet

Servings: 4
Preparation time: 40 minutes
Cook time: 40-50 minutes

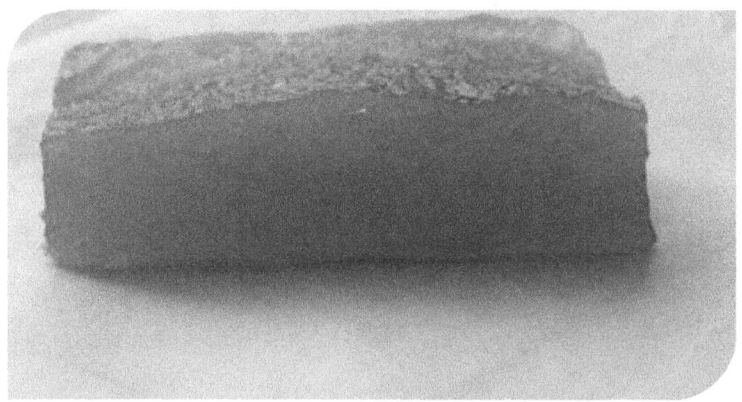

Ingredients

- *Quince pulp 1 lb. (already peeled and cored)*
- *1 lb. sugar*

Steps to Cook

1. Wash the quinces well, put them in a large pot and cover with water. Once the water starts to boil, lower the heat and cook for 45 minutes.
2. After the time, remove the quinces from the water, let cool until they do not burn, peel them, remove the heart and cut the pulp into pieces.
3. Arrange the pieces in a saucepan next to the sugar and bring to the fire. Little by little the sugar will be integrated into the pulp of the quince; after about 10 minutes you will see that the sugar is completely dissolved: at that moment grind with the mixer and cook for about 40 more minutes.
4. After the time has passed, to shape the homemade quince, we pour the quince jelly onto the container you have chosen and distribute it well; Cover with plastic wrap and take to the fridge overnight.

Nutritional Information:

- Calorie: 52
- Protein: 0.3g
- Fat: 0g
- Carbohydrates: 14g

Oat And Banana Cookies

Servings: 4
Preparation time: 10 minutes
Cook time: 15-20 minutes

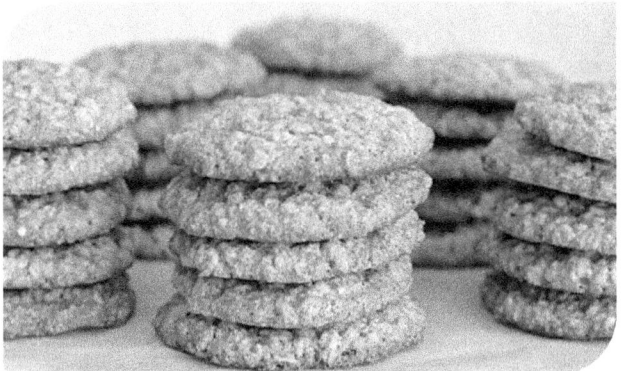

Ingredients

- 3 ripe bananas
- 1 and a half glass of oatmeal
- Chocolate chips (to taste)
- 1 tablespoon brown sugar

Steps to Cook

1. Preheat the oven to 360°F, heat up and down.
2. Cut the three bananas into slices and arrange them in a bowl, with the handle of a mortar crush the bananas well.
3. Next add the oats, chocolate chips and a tablespoon of brown sugar, knead well until a ball form.
4. Form small balls and crush lightly, put the cookies on a suitable dish for oven and bake for 15 - 20 minutes.
5. After the time, remove the cookies from the oven and let them warm on a rack.

Nutritional Information:

- Calorie: 34.1
- Protein: 1g
- Fat: 0.4g
- Carbohydrates: 7.2g

Orange and Chocolate Cake

Servings: 2
Preparation time: 1h minutes
Cook time: 455 minutes

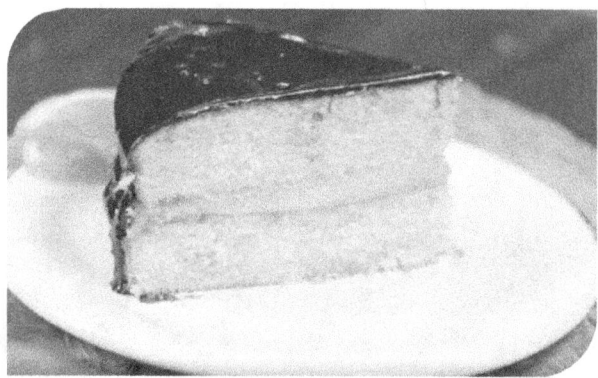

Ingredients

For the Cake:
- 3 cups of flour
- 2 cups butter
- 2 tsp. baking powder
- 2 cups of sugar
- a pinch of salt
- 2 ½ tbsp. orange zest
- 1 ½ tbsp. lemon zest
- 5 eggs
- 1 ½ cups orange juice.

For the filling:
- 1 cup of sugar
- 2 ½ tbsp. Of flour
- 1 cup orange juice
- 2 egg yolks
- 2 tbsp. of butter

Steps to Cook

1. Beat the butter, orange zest, lemon and sugar.
2. Add the eggs and gradually integrate the flour, baking powder and salt, alternating with the orange juice.
3. Flour and butter 2 molds of the same size. Distribute the mixture evenly in the two molds and bake for 45 minutes. Unmold and let cool. For the filling, in a saucepan mix the sugar, flour, orange juice and yolks. Heat over low heat and stir until it boils slightly and thickens.
4. Remove from the heat, add the butter and let cool.
5. Put one layer of cake, filling, the other layer of cake and more filling.

Nutritional Information:

- Calorie: 168.1
- Protein: 3.1g
- Fat: 11.9g
- Carbohydrates: 13.8g

Vegan Kefir

Servings: 4
Preparation time: 15 minutes

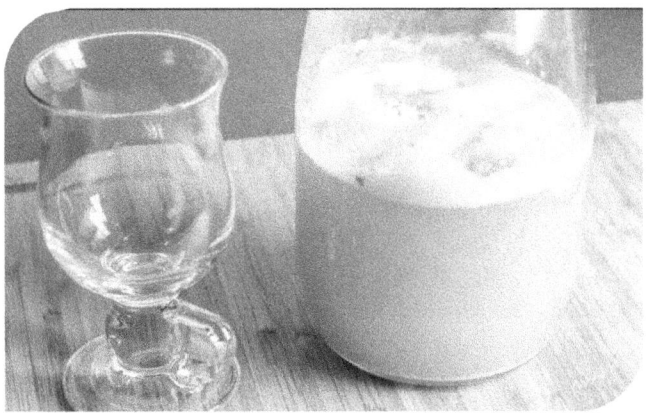

Ingredients

- 4 ¼ cup of filtered drinking water
- 5 tbsp of water kefir nodules
- 1 ½ oz. of raisins
- 5 tbsp of muscobo sugar
- 1 apple

Steps to Cook

1. In a liter of drinking water, dissolve 3 tablespoons of sugar; squeeze the juice of half a lemon (cut that half of the squeezed lemon and add it to the water), 5 tablespoons of nodules and 1 handful of raisins. Stir with a wooden spoon (do not use metal). Cover with a canvas and let stand 12 hours at room temperature. At 12 o'clock stir carefully again and cover again. 12 hours later strain the liquid. Wash the nodules and store in the refrigerator.

Nutritional Information:

- Calorie: 110
- Protein: 11g
- Fat: 0g
- Carbohydrates: 12g

Azteca Cake

Servings: 2
Preparation time: 15 minutes
Cook time: 30-40 minutes

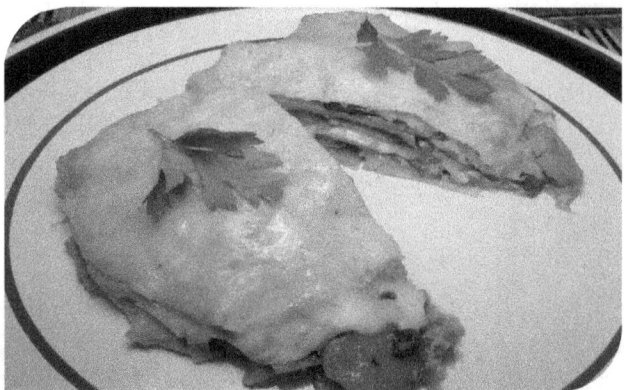

Ingredients

- 1 lb. shredded chicken supreme
- 5 chilies from heaven
- 2 cloves of garlic
- ¼ onion
- 3 cups. of water
- 8 wheat tortillas
- 1 cup corn kernels
- ½ cup cream
- 2 tbsp. chopped coriander
- 1 ½ cup of mozzarella or cheese of preference
- Salt oil

Steps to Cook

1. Heat the chilies, garlic, and onion with 3 cups of water.
2. Boil 10m. Transfer to a blender and blend with the same cooking juice.
3. Strain and reserve the sauce.
4. Brown the tortillas in oil and reserve. Dip it in the sauce and arrange in the base of an ovenproof dish.
5. Sprinkle a little shredded chicken, some corn kernels, a little of the chili sauce, cream and coriander.
6. Repeat this operation until you finish with all the ingredients.
7. Gratin in the oven at 400°F until the cheese is gratin.

Nutritional Information:

- Calorie: 140
- Protein: 11g
- Fat: 12g
- Carbohydrates: 10g

Strawberry Milkshake

Servings: 1-2
Preparation time: 5 minutes

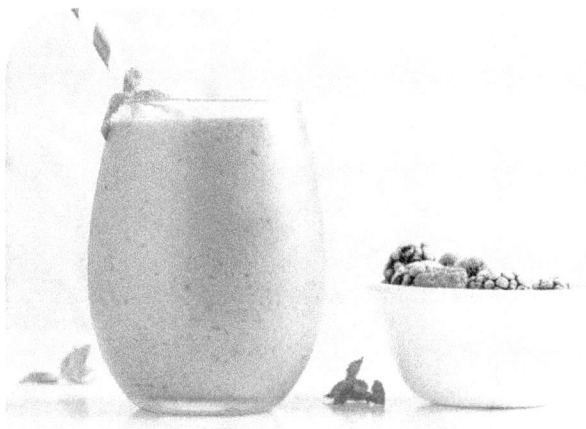

Ingredients

- ½ lb. strawberry
- 2 strawberry soy yogurts
- 1 cup of soy milk
- 4 cookies without ingredients of animal origin
- 2 tbsp of sugar

Steps to Cook

1. Clean the strawberries and put them in the blender glass together with the yogurts, sugar and milk. You can use the yogurt cups to measure the milk, filled the same ones and add that amount. When it is well mixed, break the cookies and add them. Continue beating until everything is homogeneous and ready. You can leave it a little in the fridge so that it is very cold.

Nutritional Information:

- Calorie: 640
- Protein: 12g
- Fat: 22g
- Carbohydrates: 101g

Potato and Mushroom Cake

Servings: 8
Preparation time: 20 minutes
Cook time: 1h

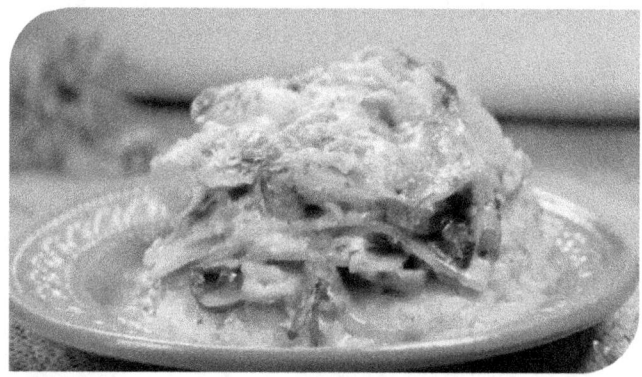

Ingredients

- 8 medium potatoes
- ½ lb. of mushroom
- ½ lb. of portobello in thin sheets
- 1 cup of grated gruyere
- ½ cup grated Parmesan
- 3 tbsp. parsley
- 1 tbsp. oregano
- ½ cup vegetable broth
- salt, pepper and nutmeg
- 1 tbsp. butter

Steps to Cook

1. Heat the oven to 360°F and grease a baking dish with the tablespoon of butter
2. Cut the potatoes and mushrooms into very thin sheets
3. In the greased refractory make layers of potatoes, mushrooms, gruyere, seasoning between layers.
4. At the end add the vegetable stock, cover with aluminum and bake for 1h.
5. Uncover, cover with cheese and gratin with Parmesan until golden.

Nutritional Information:

- Calorie: 117.5
- Protein: 2.9g
- Fat: 3.2g
- Carbohydrates: 20.2g

Oat Milk

Servings: 1-2
Preparation time: 5 minutes
Cook time: 15 minutes

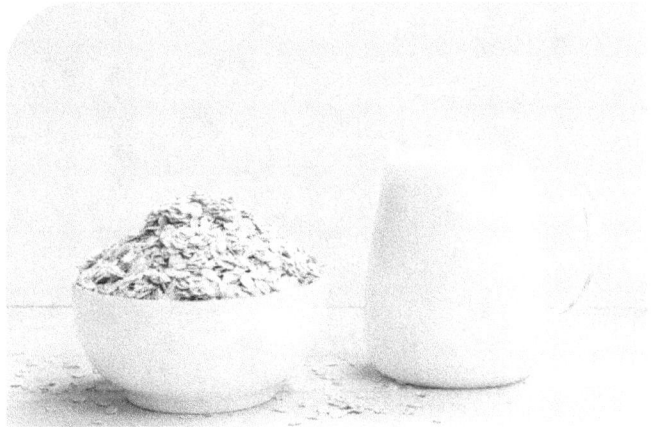

Ingredients

- ½ cup rolled whole oats
- 3 cups of water
- 2 tsp maple syrup
- ½ tsp vanilla extract
- Ta tsp of sea salt

Steps to Cook

1. Mix the oats, water, maple syrup, vanilla, and salt in a blender and mix for 30 seconds.
2. Place the fine mesh strainer over a large bowl and strain the milk without pushing excess pulp through the strainer. This will create a creamier texture that is not gritty or sticky.
3. Add more maple syrup, to taste, if desired. Let cool overnight. but if you want to take it once prepared, put an ice on it. It is much tastier fresh.

Nutritional Information:

- Calorie: 120
- Protein: 3g
- Fat: 5g
- Carbohydrates: 16g

Strawberry Biscuit Cake

Servings: 4
Preparation time: 15 minutes
Cook time: 30-40 minutes

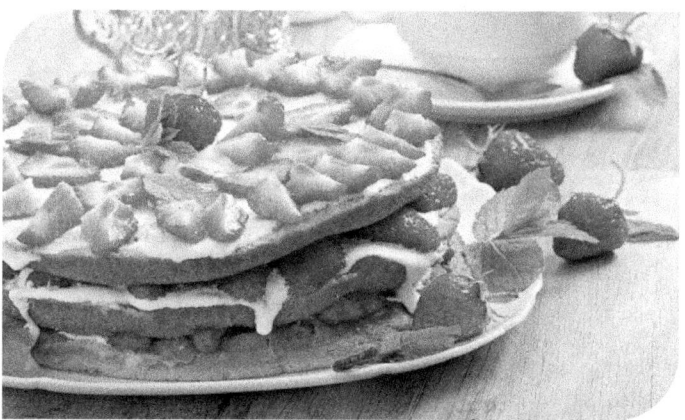

Ingredients

- 1 can of condensed milk
- ½ cup milk
- 4 egg yolks
- 1 tablet of semi-bitter chocolate
- 1 pot of cream
- ½ lb. of cookies
- 1 cup of whipping cream
- ½ lb. sliced strawberries

Steps to Cook

1. Place the milk, condensed milk and egg yolks over low heat, stirring constantly until thick. Cool for 1 hour.
2. In a bowl, mix the melted chocolate with the cream. Reserve.
3. On a platter, put the condensed milk mixture, a large number of cookies on top, then the chocolate mixture, the second portion of wafers and cover with the whipping cream.
4. Finish the preparation with strawberry slices on top. Arrange in circular shapes.
5. Enjoy it!

Nutritional Information:

- Calorie: 90
- Protein: 2.3g
- Fat: 2.7g
- Carbohydrates: 15.3g

Red Fruit Shake

Servings: 1-2
Preparation time: 5 minutes

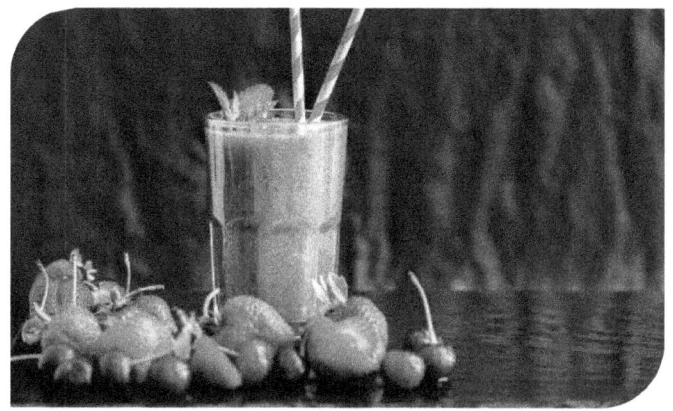

Ingredients

- ½ lb. of strawberries
- ½ lb. raspberries
- ½ lb. of blackberries
- ½ cup of water
- Agave syrup (optional)
- Flax or chia seeds (optional)

Steps to Cook

1. First wash the fruits well. Cut the strawberries too, but if they are not very large, it is not necessary.
2. Put the fruits in the base of the mixer and crush until you have a smooth and homogeneous texture.
3. Raspberries and frozen blackberries give a very creamy texture and also makes the smoothie super cool. If you use them frozen, keep in mind the type of mixer you use, if it is not very powerful; better take them out of the freezer a few minutes before so they are not too hard.
4. You can also add some seeds, flax or chia, crushing them at the same time as the fruits and you will provide extra nutrients.

Nutritional Information:

- Calorie: 130
- Protein: 1g
- Fat: 0g
- Carbohydrates: 31g

Oreo Crepes Tower

Servings: 8
Preparation time: 25 minutes
Cook time: 40 minutes

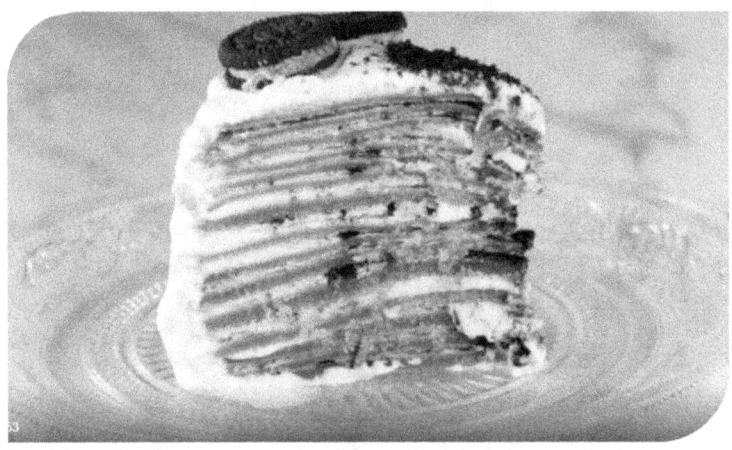

Ingredients

- 1 cup flour
- 2 tbsp. cocoa powder
- 4 tbsp. of sugar
- 2 eggs
- 2 tbsp. melted butter
- 1 cup milk
- 1⅓ cup heavy cream
- ¼ cup sugar
- 1 tsp. vanilla essence
- 7 crushed Oreo cookies

Steps to Cook

1. Mix all the ingredients for the pancakes.
2. Make 15 pancakes.
3. Separate the cream from the Oreo and crush them.
4. Make the pancake tower sandwiching with the whipped cream and the crushed Oreo.
5. Decorate with whipped cream and mini-Oreos.

Nutritional Information:

- Calorie: 121.1
- Protein: 3.4g
- Fat: 6.5g
- Carbohydrates: 15.7g

Coriander And Walnut Pesto

Servings: 2
Preparation time: 5 minutes

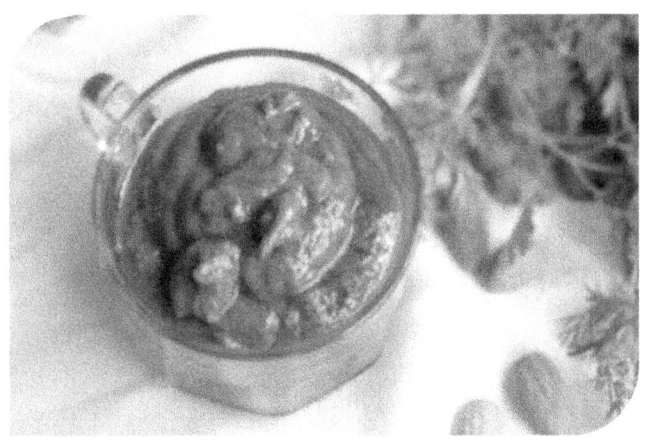

Ingredients

- 1 coriander bundle
- 2 cloves of garlic
- 1 handful of walnuts
- Oil to taste

Steps to Cook

1. Blend coriander, garlic, salt and walnuts with a little oil to form a paste.
2. Add oil little by little. Store in glass jars and refrigerate in the refrigerator.

Nutritional Information:

- Calorie: 35
- Protein: 0g
- Fat: 4g
- Carbohydrates: 0g

Hazelnut Milk With Cocoa

Servings: 2
Preparation time: 5 minutes

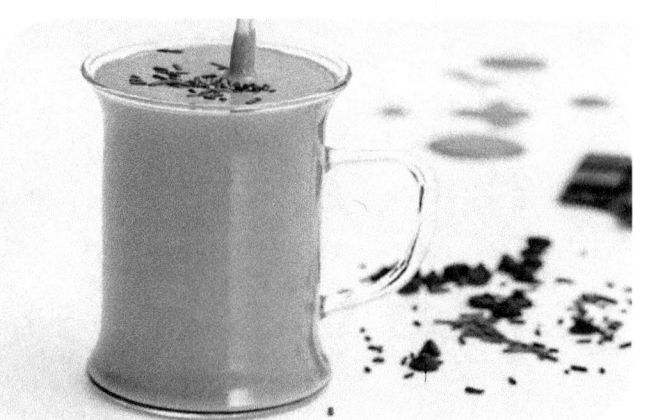

Ingredients

- 4 cups of water
- 3 ½ oz. hazelnuts
- 1 tbsp of cocoa

Steps to Cook

1. Put in the glass of the vegan milker 1 liter of warm water and in the filter 3 ½ oz. of hazelnuts. Crush for one minute with an arm mixer. Add the cocoa and crush again until it mixes well.
2. In case that you have not made the milk and you are not using the pulp if not directly the hazelnuts, add a teaspoon of hazelnut milk (or another vegetable).

Nutritional Information:

- Calorie: 169
- Protein: 3g
- Fat: 10g
- Carbohydrates: 14g

Tofu Cream: Spreadable Tofu Cheese

Servings: 2
Preparation time: 5 minutes

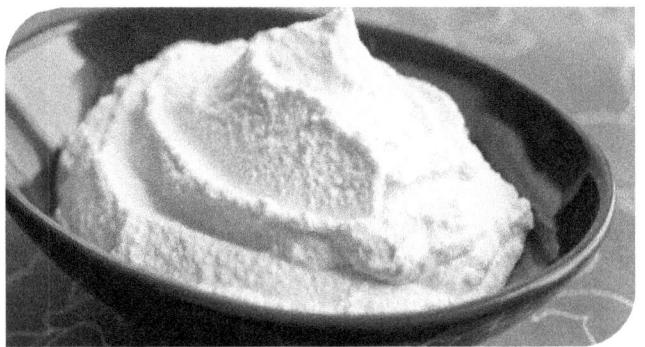

Ingredients

- ¼ lb. tofu
- 1 tbsp titanium nutritional yeast
- 1 tbsp of lemon juice
- Neutral oil
- Neutral vegan milk or water

Steps to Cook

1. Mix everything well. add oil little by little until it becomes consistent.
2. Add if necessary, vegan milk or water to lighten.
3. Store in a plate in the refrigerator.

Nutritional Information:

- Calorie: 159.3
- Protein: 5g
- Fat: 4.5g
- Carbohydrates: 23.7g

Almond Milk

Servings: 2
Preparation time: 8 h

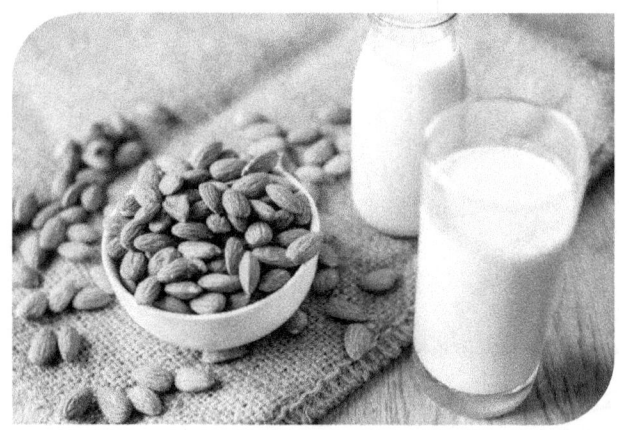

Ingredients

- 100g raw almonds
- 1 liter of water

Steps to Cook

1. Put the liter of water in the transparent glass, put the previously soaked almonds for about 8 hours in the filter and crush with a hand mixer for one minute at maximum power.
2. Drain well and store the milk in the fridge, which lasts about 3 days.

Nutritional Information:

- Calorie: 39
- Protein: 1g
- Fat: 3g
- Carbohydrates: 3.5g

Ginger Milk

Servings: 2
Preparation time: 5 minutes
Cook time: 5-10 minutes

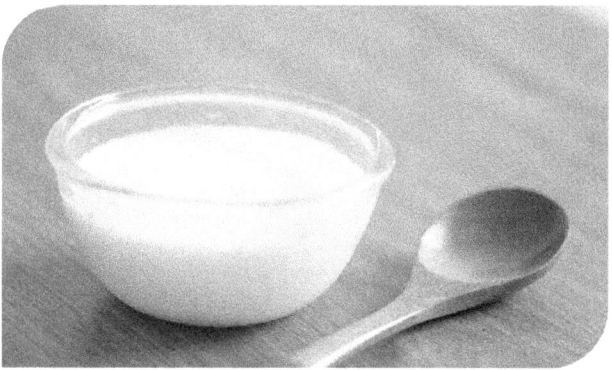

Ingredients

- 1 ½ cup of vegetable milk
- Grated or powdered ginger
- Pinch of salt
- Muscovy sugar

Steps to Cook

1. Heat all ingredients in a saucepan over medium low heat. Stir well until it boils.
2. Serve and enjoy!

Nutritional Information:

- Calorie: 200
- Protein: 8g
- Fat: 10g
- Carbohydrates: 20g

Fresh Mint And Basil Ice Cream

Servings: 4
Preparation time: 5 minutes

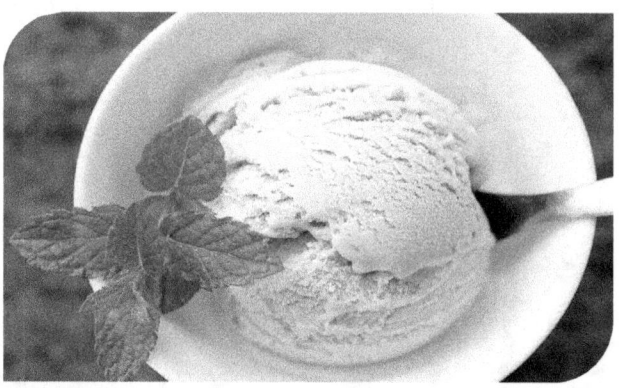

Ingredients

- ½ lb. raw cashews
- 1 lb. peeled and diced pears
- 1 ¾ oz. white raisins
- 3 ½ oz. fresh basil leaves
- 3 ½ oz. fresh mint leaves
- 1 ½ oz. of water (enough to mix)

Steps to Cook

1. Soak the cashews in water for about 12 hours and then remove the water.
2. Put all the ingredients in a blender and blend until you get a uniform and homogeneous cream.
3. If you have an ice cream maker, you can put the mix in it to finish the ice cream. If you don't have this machine, just put the mix in the freezer until it has a harder consistency.

Nutritional Information:

- Calorie: 247
- Protein: 5g
- Fat: 16g
- Carbohydrates: 23g

Watermelon Smoothie

Servings: 4
Preparation time: 5 minutes

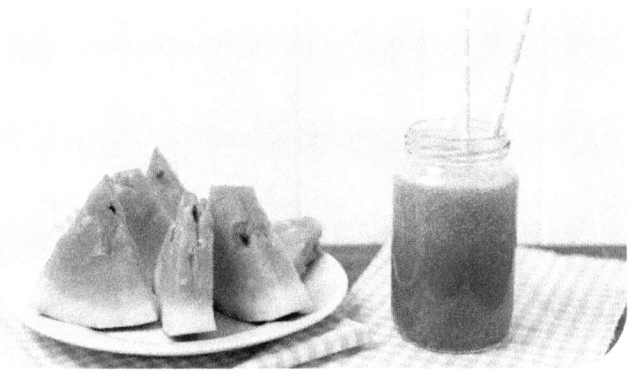

Ingredients

- 1 lb. of watermelon
- 1 soy yogurt
- 2 glasses of crushed ice

Steps to Cook

1. The preparation of this watermelon smoothie is very simple; you just have to put the glass of the blender the watermelon cut into pieces and the soy yogurt. Whisk until well mixed and watermelon completely melts. A fairly liquid and homogeneous mixture will remain.
2. To finish the smoothie, you just have to add the ice and beat again so that it melts.
3. Let's enjoy it!

Nutritional Information:

- Calorie: 113.5
- Protein: 4.3g
- Fat: 1.7g
- Carbohydrates: 22.1g

Banana Puccino

Servings: 4
Preparation time: 5 minutes

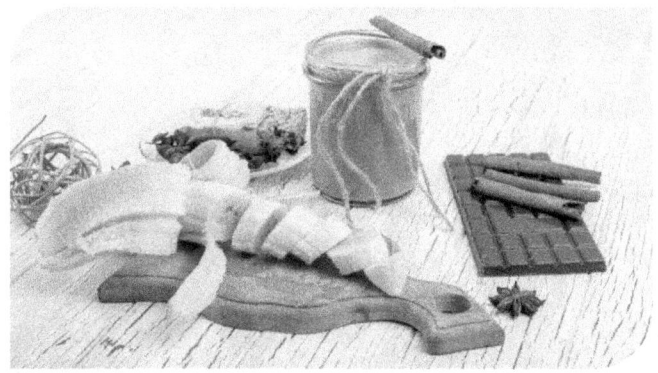

Ingredients

- 2 cups vegan milk
- ½ banana
- ½ cup of pure coffee
- 3 dates (pitted)
- ½ tsp cocoa powder
- ½ tsp cinnamon

Steps to Cook

1. Blend everything. If it is necessary and you want to make it sweeter, add mascabo or more dates. You can also add nutmeg or vanilla.

Nutritional Information:

- Calorie: 105
- Protein: 1.3g
- Fat: 0.4g
- Carbohydrates: 27g

Vegan Potato Cheese

Servings: 5
Preparation time: 5 minutes
Cook time: 10-15 minutes

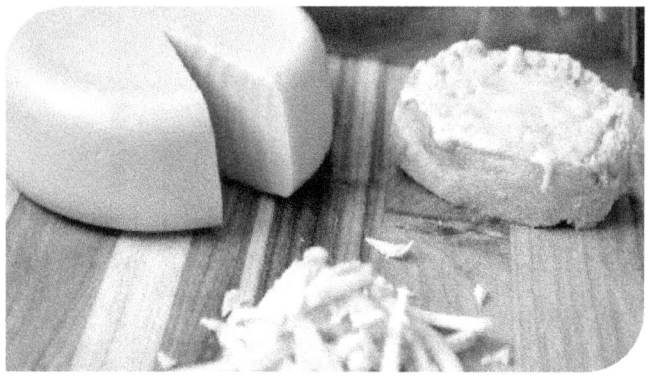

Ingredients

- 2 potatoes
- 1 tbsp nutritional yeast
- Pepper
- Oil

Steps to Cook

1. Cook the potatoes.
2. Let them cool.
3. Process everything together with the rest of the ingredients.
4. Store in an airtight container in the refrigerator.

Nutritional Information:

- Calorie: 94
- Protein: 2.2g
- Fat: 7g
- Carbohydrates: 6.3g

Purple smoothie

Servings: 5
Preparation time: 5 minutes

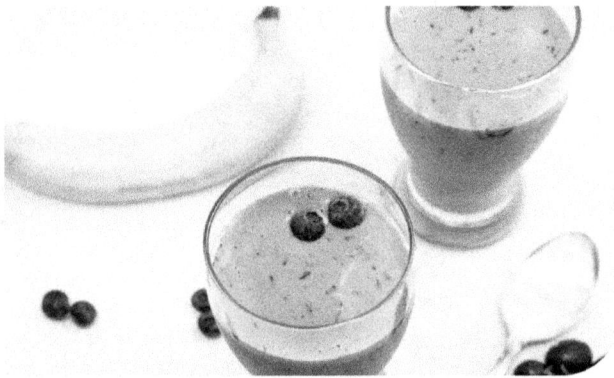

Ingredients

- 1 frozen banana, sliced
- 1 tsp of açaí powder (or in pulp)
- ½ cup frozen cranberries
- 1 prickly pear or kiwi
- 1 fresh banana, sliced
- grated coconut

Steps to Cook

1. Processing the banana and the açaí powder or if you get it in the pulp is the same.
2. Add the frozen blueberries.
3. On top, garnish with prickly pear or kiwi, banana slices and grated coconut.
4. Enjoy.

Nutritional Information:

- Calorie: 140
- Protein: 1g
- Fat: 0g
- Carbohydrates: 33g

Coffee Truffles

Servings: 5
Preparation time: 5 minutes

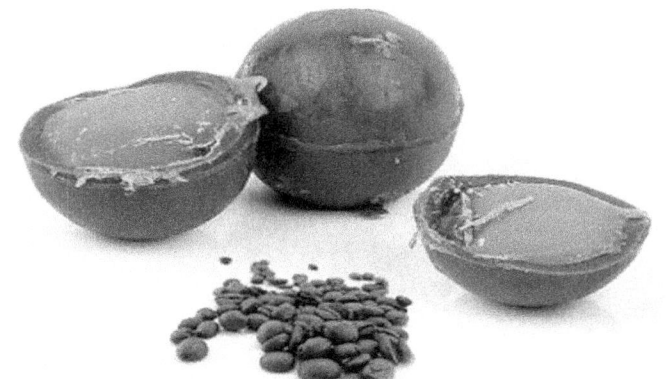

Ingredients

- ¾ lb. sweet sponge cake crumbs or vanilla
- ½ cup boiling water
- 2 tbsp instant coffee
- 10 dates
- 1 tbsp vanilla
- 3 ½ oz. dark chocolate
- Toppings at ease

Steps to Cook

1. Crumble the cake and add the coffee dissolved in the boiling water. Work with a fork until the entire crumb is moist.
2. Process the dates in a mixer or kitchen robot with a little water to help the process. Add part of the crumb and vanilla and continue processing until well-integrated.
3. Add this mixture to the rest of the crumb and integrate with a fork.
4. With your hands slightly damp, form balls until the mixture is finished and take to the fridge for at least 2 hours so that they are firm.
5. Pass the balls through melted chocolate or any other bath you want.
6. Store in an airtight bottle in the fridge for up to 5 days.

Nutritional Information:

- Calorie: 111
- Protein: 2.1g
- Fat: 11.9g
- Carbohydrates: 6.1g

Vegan Corn Cake

Servings: 5
Preparation time: 5 minutes
Cook time: 30-40 minutes

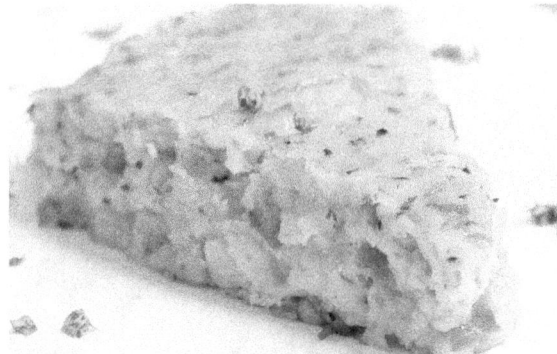

Ingredients

- Vegan cake batter
- 1 small onion
- 1 small bell pepper
- Margarine to taste
- 2 tbsp cornstarch
- Soy milk to taste
- 2 cans of yellow corn kernels
- Pepper
- Nutmeg

Steps to Cook

1. Chop the onion and the bell pepper and fry them in a saucepan with the margarine, until they are soft.
2. Add the corn starch and mix well.
3. Incorporate the soy milk and continue cooking until a thick béchamel is formed.
4. Turn off the heat, season and add the nutmeg.
5. Add the drained corn grains to the preparation and mix well.
6. Spread the tart dough in a tart pan and fill with the preparation. if the dough is bought, cover with the other dough cover.
7. Add a little margarine or oil and take to a moderate oven until cooked.

Nutritional Information:

- Calorie: 67.1
- Protein: 1.8g
- Fat: 0.6g
- Carbohydrates: 15.2g

Vegan Cocoa Muffins

Servings: 2-4
Preparation time: 15 minutes
Cook time: 20 minutes

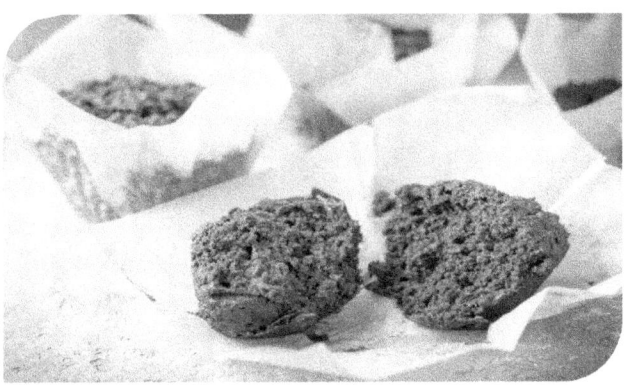

Ingredients

- ½ lb. of whole wheat flour
- ¼ lb. of whole cane sugar
- 3 tsp baking powder
- 1 tbsp of soy flour dissolved in water
- 1 cup of soy milk
- ¼ cup of sunflower oil
- 3-4 tablespoons cocoa powder

Steps to Cook

1. In a large bowl mix the flour, sugar and yeast.
2. In a jug mix the milk and oil. in a glass dissolve the soy flour in a little water and add it to the jar mixture.
3. Mix this liquid with the flour mixture and mix well.
4. Fill the mixture with papers or cupcake molds and bake.

Nutritional Information:

- Calorie: 197.7
- Protein: 2.6g
- Fat: 10.3g
- Carbohydrates: 25g

Vegan Chocolate Peanut Butter Cheesecake

Servings: 4-6
Preparation time: 15 minutes
Cook time: 20-30 minutes

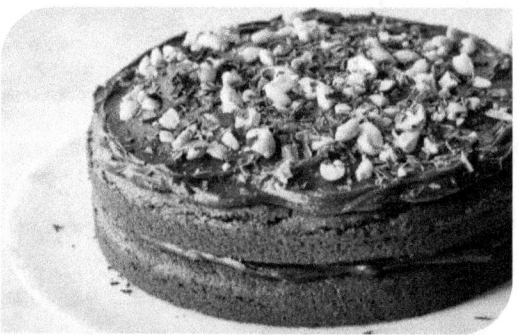

Ingredients

For the base:
- 3 ½ oz. dates
- 3 ½ oz. of raisins
- 3 ½ oz. of sunflower seeds
- 1 ½ oz. of walnuts
- 3 ½ oz. of peanuts

filling:
- ½ lb. of tofu
- 3 ½ oz. of cocoa
- 2 oz. of muscabo sugar
- 3 ½ oz. of coconut oil
- 2 oz. coconut milk
- Pinch of salt

Steps to Cook

1. Process the dates, raisins, sunflower, walnuts, peanuts and cocoa and assemble the base of the cake.
2. Spread with peanut butter. Blend the tofu, cocoa, sugar, and coconut oil, 50g of peanut butter, coconut milk, salt and vanilla essence.
3. Decorate with melted chocolate.

Nutritional Information:

- Calorie: 197.7
- Protein: 2.6g
- Fat: 10.3g
- Carbohydrates: 25g

Vegan Chocolate Pudding

Servings: 2-4
Preparation time: 10 minutes
Cook time: 45 minutes

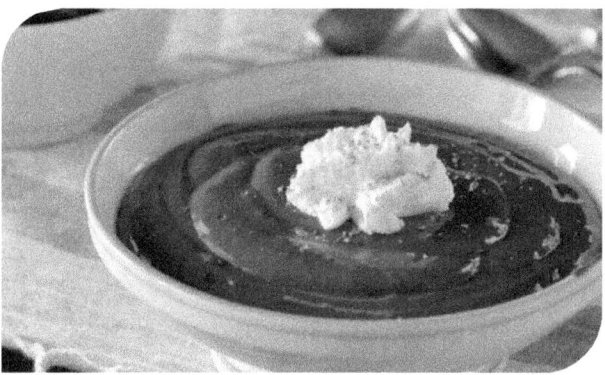

Ingredients

- 2 cups organic wheat flour
- 1 tablespoon baking powder
- ½ cup organic cocoa
- 1 cup oil
- 1 cup organic sugar
- Zest of 1 orange
- Pinch of salt
- Juice of 1 orange
- 1 cup vegan milk

Steps to Cook

1. Mix the sugar and the oil.
2. Add the vegan milk and continue mixing.
3. Add the pinch of salt, zest and orange juice.
4. Sift the dry ones and incorporate with an enveloping movement.
5. Cook in an oven at 170ºC until a toothpick is inserted and it comes out moist.

Nutritional Information:

- Calorie: 197.7
- Protein: 2.6g
- Fat: 10.3g
- Carbohydrates: 25g

21 Day meal plan for Plant-based Diet

You may be a bit skeptical and think that it is impossible to lose weight in 3 weeks. However, it is possible. It is just a matter of going to the doctor and the nutritionist and starting to follow their instructions while improving your lifestyle in general - and in the process, you learn to maintain them in a consistent way - little by little.

Keep in mind that there is no magic formula to lose weight in a short time and those that claim to be, only manage to put your health at risk. Therefore, it is important that you always follow what your doctor and nutritionist tell you.

On the other hand, keep in mind that each organism is different and what may be "good" for one may not work for the other at all. This is the reason why you should avoid following dietary advice and recommendations from third parties (family, friends, co-workers, etc.) or people through social networks.

Day 1

Write your goals in a notebook or paper and leave them in a visible place. Start with a simple exercise routine (for example, going for a walk).

Day 2

Eliminate sources of liquid calories, namely coffee with sugar, soda, and alcohol. Replace them with water, green tea, and natural fruit juices. Write what you eat on a sheet without forgetting anything. Keep in mind that alcohol has been shown to increase the risk of getting sick, beyond affecting body composition.

Day 3

Take the second day of training. You can increase your walking distance, intensity, or add another exercise. According to a study published in Obesity Reviews, interval exercises are the best to stimulate weight loss.

Day 4

Change from 3 large meals to 6 small meals each day. Don't forget to add fruits, vegetables, fiber, and protein to all snacks.

Day 5

Make a shopping list with healthy foods and go to the market with it, without adding anything else. If you could not resist the temptation, it would be good if you discarded, gave away, or even sold the products that you are not allowed to consume.

Day 6

Weigh yourself and write down the kilos in the notebook. Pick an activity to do at least 3 times a week. It can be a sport, a dance class, or going out to exercise in a park.

Day 7

Plan the diet for the following week and, if necessary, make another purchase at a fruit, vegetable, and vegetable fair, or at a neighborhood store that has these types of items. This type of environment has fresh and seasonal foods that invite you to acquire what is best for the body.

Day 8

Continue with your exercise plan. You can hire a coach or change the exercises yourself so as not to get bored.

Day 9

Add to your diet fruit and a vegetable that you have never eaten before or that you have not enjoyed for a long time. Try to eat them raw or steamed. If you like it, you can find other healthy ways to eat it to integrate it into your diet whenever you want, but without falling into monotony.

Day 10

Eliminate sources of trans fats from your diet and don't forget to exercise. These lipids are capable of increasing inflammation, according to a study published in Progress in Lipid Research. This leads to a worsening of metabolic health.

Day 11

Make sure you are drinking enough water, as long as your body requires.

Day 12

Pay attention to the number of fibers you consume per day. At least 35 grams is recommended. If you don't reach this number, eat a handful of almonds.

Day 13

Count the calories you consumed the previous days based on the intake chart. Check how much is the minimum and maximum allowed according to your age, weight, and height, as well as the goal of kilos you want to eliminate.

Day 14

Plan your diet for the following week by shopping and analyzing the foods you have at home. Eat more fruits in season.

Day 15

Change the physical activity you were doing so far or increase the difficulty. You can add more weight, reduce marks, or walk longer. You can also add a new set or more exercises to the routine.

Day 16

Follow a new food cooking technique in relation to what you have been doing. It can be, for example, steamed or grilled. Try to eat more raw and fat-free menus.

Day 17

Eat less dinner than the previous days and look for a different protein source than usual. For example, if you usually eat chicken or tuna, switch to meat or salmon.

Day 18

Train a little more than the previous session. Check the loads, times, or distances and try adding new exercises.

Day 19

Review your goals and see if you are close to reaching your goal. You can weigh yourself or try on clothes from the previous season that you did not fit before starting this 21-day plan to lose weight.

Day 20

Make the purchase for the following days. At this point you will not want to go back to the routine you had three weeks before, because you will look slimmer, but also with more energy and vitality.

Day 21

Be more precise in your vision and analyze the changes you have made in your life. Strengthen your commitment. Keep going. You have already created your healthy habit!

What can you eat within your 21-day plan?

"What can I eat?" It is a common question among those who want to lose weight in a healthy way and without starving. That is because they want to know the alternatives to begin to re-educate themselves in terms of food and thus add steps to reach their goal.

Some of the options would be the following that we are going to share with you.

Breakfast and snack

The foods allowed in the 21-day plan are as follows:

- Raisins
- Fruits
- Oats
- Skimmed cream cheese
- 1 cup of milk (250 ml)
- 3 cookies without salt or sugar
- 2 slices of whole wheat bread
- 1 slice of low-fat cheese
- 1 teaspoon of sweetener (5 ml)

Lunch and dinner

A bowl of soup is consumed as a starter. The main dish is a small piece of meat with cooked vegetables and a side of salad. For dessert we will have a fruit.

- Light gelatin
- Leafy vegetable
- Lemon juice
- Olive oil
- Nonfat yogurt
- Apple vinager
- Dry pasta (not stuffed)
- Homemade vegetable soup
- Natural juices without sugar
- Raw or steamed vegetables
- Legumes (lentils, chickpeas, beans)
- Brown rice, quinoa, barley, millet, or wheat
- Seasonings (ground garlic, cloves, turmeric)
- Aromatic herbs (basil, rosemary, thyme).
- Raw fruits for dessert (strawberries, peach, orange)

Conclusion

As we explained at the beginning, the integral plant-based diet restricts the consumption of any type of processed food, they are only accepted in their integral and whole state, and that is the great difference with the vegan diet.

Although this name may seem to suggest that with this diet we can only eat plants, the truth is that it is something broader, it refers to having a more plant-based diet and reducing the consumption of products of animal origin.

Thus, within this new food method, the following foods can be consumed:

- Vegetables
- Vegetables.Fruits
- Grains (chickpeas, lentils, adzuki beans)
- Cereals (brown rice, quinoa, millet, buckwheat, etc)
- Nuts, Seeds, Legumes

And, yes, to get a healthy diet what you have to choose is to choose that these foods are as less processed as possible. That is, the equation is simple: increase fruits and vegetables to the detriment of meats and fish, mainly.

Improve your health

Scientific articles that show the benefits of increasing the consumption of plant-based foods.

Articles that tell us that following a more plant-based diet helps prevent and even reverse some of the diseases that cause more incidences of deaths in the Western world, being in many situations more effective than medication or surgical interventions. This type of diet is the only one that has been shown to reverse the number 1 cause of death: heart attacks.

Changing some lifestyle habits (moving the body at least 30 min / day) can reverse cardiovascular diseases.

Helps prevent certain types of cancer, reduces the incidence of heart disease and diabetes, cholesterol, hypertension, Alzheimer's, Parkinson's, rheumatoid arthritis, ulcers and infections.

It has a positive effect on the prevention of abdominal fat accumulation, the appearance of acne, aging, allergies, asthma, body odor, cellulite, eczema, metabolic syndrome and control of body weight.

Maintain your proper weight

The accumulation of weight that one is adding over the years, so to prevent the appearance of both, following a plant diet will be our ally.

Reduces obesity: it is a diet that is very low in saturated fat and, therefore, will activate the metabolism and avoid disorders such as overweight or obesity.

Improves intestinal transit: and another benefit is that a plant-based diet is very rich in fiber. This nutrient helps us regulate intestinal transit, improve digestive function and avoid discomforts such as flatulence, bloating, constipation, etc.

For ecology, environmental benefits

- It reduces the emission of greenhouse gases, the consumption of a diet that includes meat, creates 7 times more greenhouse gases compared to a plant diet.
- Reduces the emission of methane gas produced by animals.
- Reduces fossil fuel consumption. 1 calorie from animal protein requires 11 times more fossil fuel to produce.
- Reduces the use of water worldwide. Most of the water worldwide is used in meat production factories. It takes more than 2,400 gallons of water to produce 453 grams of meat, while only 25 gallons are required to produce the same amount of wheat.
- Reduces the use of land area. The production of meat for human use uses 30% of the earth's surface.
- Reduce deforestation. Forests are deforested to produce grains to later feed livestock. An equivalent of 7 soccer fields are deforested every minute worldwide. Extending the "plant-based diet" to the western population would not only improve human health.

For all these reasons and many more, we encourage you to switch to a plant-based diet for at least one day can help you see how a change in your diet can be a new beginning for a healthier and more energetic life.

www.ingramcontent.com/pod-product-compliance
Lightning Source LLC
Chambersburg PA
CBHW081506080526

44589CB00017B/2665